QUICK LOOKS

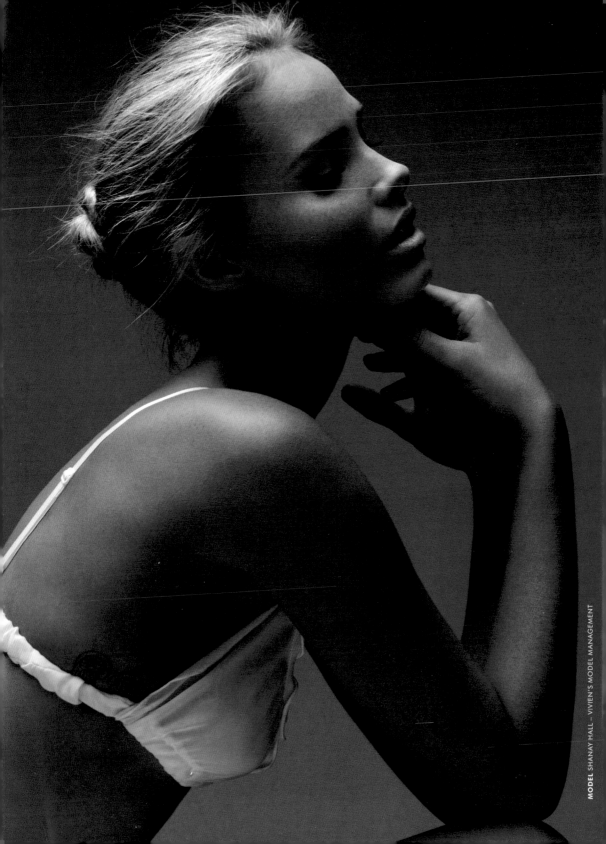

RAE MORRIS

QUICK LOOKS.

BEAUTIFUL MAKEUP IN MINUTES

Photography by Steven Chee

ARENA
ALLEN&UNWIN

First published in 2012

Copyright © Rae Morris 2012

Copyright © photography Steven Chee 2012

Arena Books, an imprint of
Allen & Unwin
Sydney, Melbourne, Auckland, London

83 Alexander Street
Crows Nest NSW 2065
Australia
Phone: (61 2) 8425 0100
Fax: (61 2) 9906 2218
Email: info@allenandunwin.com
Web: www.allenandunwin.com

Cataloguing-in-Publication details are available from
the National Library of Australia
www.trove.nla.gov.au

ISBN 978 1 74331 265 0

Design by Stephen Smedley, Tonto Design
Printed in China at Everbest Printing Co.
10 9 8 7 6 5 4 3 2 1

Front cover: Shanay Hall – Vivien's Model Management.
Hair by Heath Massi. Manicure by Belinda Johnson.
Back cover (from left to right): Caitlin Lomax –
Priscilla's Model Management, Sarah Grant – Chadwick
Models, Jenny Day – Vivien's Model Management.

CONTENTS

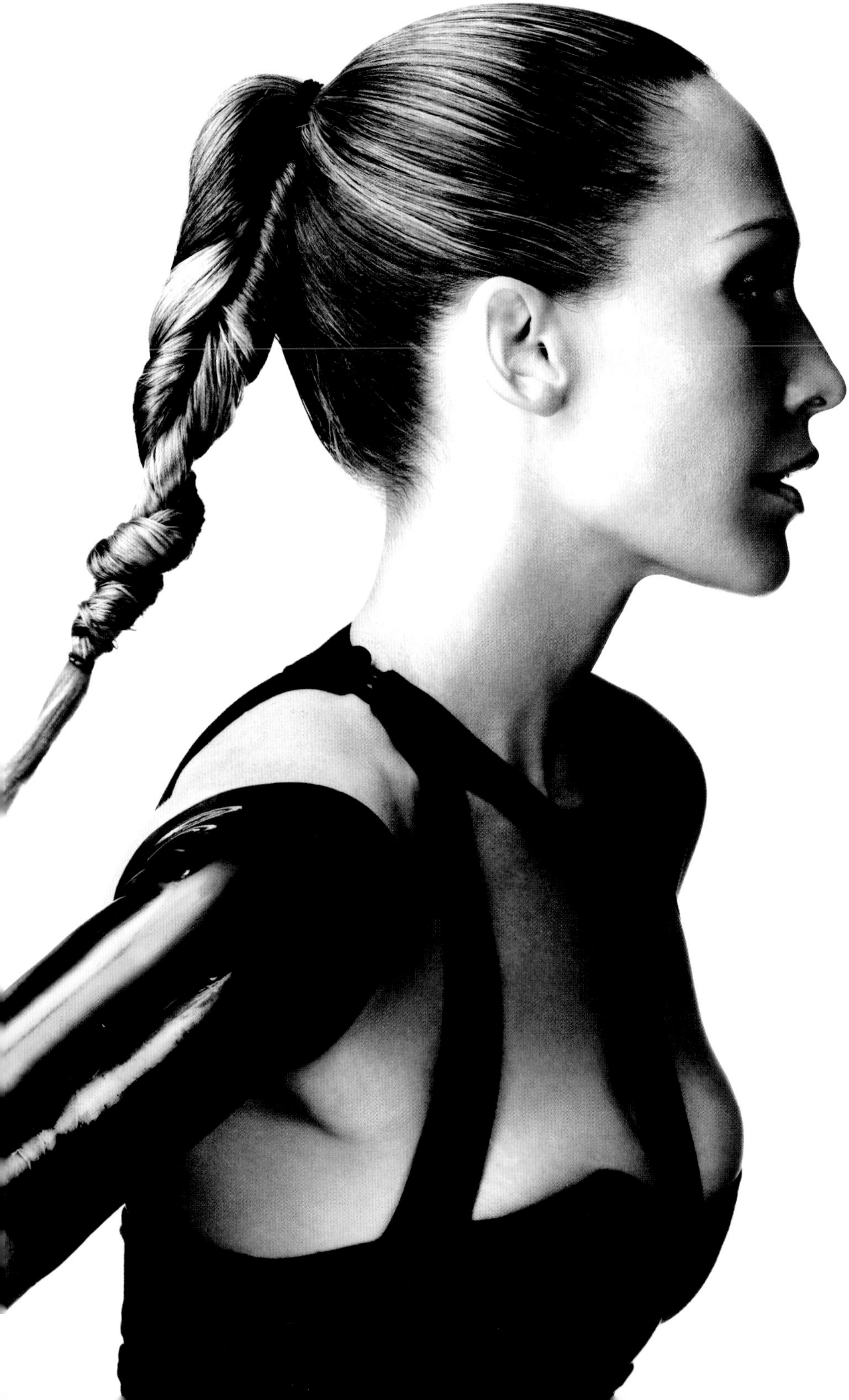

MODEL ERIKA HEYNATZ – CHIC MANAGEMENT

INTRODUCTION

A big part of my job involves working under pressure at fashion shows, where everything has to be done quickly. The tricks I've learnt over the years are the inspiration for this book, which is about creating beautiful makeup looks *fast*. Whether you have five or fifteen minutes to spare, you can use *Quick Looks* to achieve a sophisticated look for day, a chic look for a dinner date straight after work or a fabulous look for a gala evening event.

This book is also for those women who are put off by the thought of how long it takes to apply their makeup. I guarantee that even a piece of sticky tape can help make it perfect in less than a minute, while the simplest reshaping of your brow can completely transform your eye shape.

And my number one tip? If time is of the essence, always do your eyes first, because you can apply your foundation and lipstick as you're literally racing out the door.

Every woman can do her own makeup by following my expert tips and looks, all of which feature clear instructions and beautiful step-by-step photographs. Always follow the order given in each sequence, as it will increase your speed and proficiency. There are also some great tips for women over 40.

It's all about your brushes. You can do more with minimal product and an incredible brush range than with cotton buds and drawers of makeup. After using every makeup brush on the planet, I know the good ones are hard to find, so I've designed my own range. Every brush I've had made is the best of its type; I have done all the research and testing for you. You can purchase them from my website—www.raemorris.com.

To me, this book is about more than makeup—it's about how you feel about yourself, which determines how you face the world. I hope this book helps make you look and feel *fabulous*.

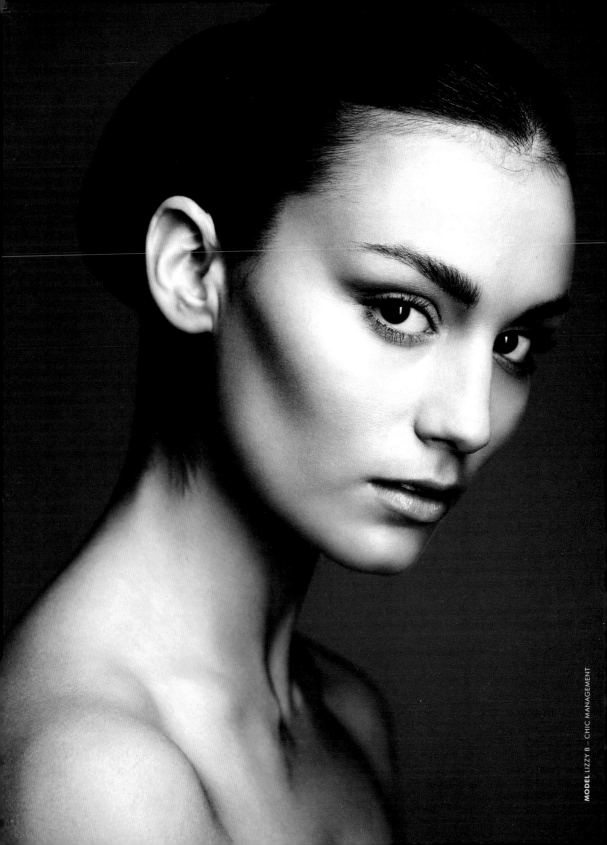

1 EXPRESS FIXES

IF YOU'RE PULLING OFF A
QUICK FIX, HERE'S MY LIST
OF ESSENTIALS AND HOW
TO USE THEM.

EXPRESS MAKEUP KIT

Use the following list as a guide to buying your makeup essentials.

Skin

- [ ] Skin scrub (bicarb soda + water-based moisturiser—see page 10)
- [ ] Moisturiser
- [ ] Primer
- [ ] Anti-shine primer
- [ ] Foundation
- [ ] Concealer
- [ ] Powder (if required)
- [ ] Highlighters
- [ ] Luminiser (if required)
- [ ] Bronzer
- [ ] Blush
- [ ] Contour cream
- [ ] Sunscreen

Eyes

- [ ] Tweezers
- [ ] Brow pencils
- [ ] Brow mascaras
- [ ] Kohl pencils (black, grey, deep brown and creamy white)
- [ ] Gel or liquid eyeliner
- [ ] Eye shadows/pigments (at least three different colours)
- [ ] Mascara
- [ ] Eyelash curlers
- [ ] False lashes
- [ ] Eyelash applicator
- [ ] Latex
- [ ] Sticky tape (for eyeliner)
- [ ] Eye drops

Lips

- [ ] Lipstick
- [ ] Lip gloss
- [ ] Lip pencil
- [ ] Lip balm

Hands

- [ ] Hand cream (also great for dry, cracked heels)
- [ ] Cuticle oil

Makeup brushes

- [ ] Brush cleaner
- [ ] Double-ended concealer brush
- [ ] Fibre-optic foundation brush/radiance brush
- [ ] Eyeliner brushes
- [ ] Combined mascara wand/angle brush
- [ ] Mini square blending brush
- [ ] Eye shadow blending brushes
- [ ] Lip brush
- [ ] Kabuki brush
- [ ] Powder brush
- [ ] Fan brush
- [ ] Disposable mascara wands (or clean the one you're about to throw out)

Other essentials

- [ ] Non-perfumed, non-alcoholic baby wipes
- [ ] Blotting papers—non-powdered
- [ ] Makeup remover
- [ ] Tissues
- [ ] Hair clips
- [ ] Cotton buds
- [ ] Manicure scissors
- [ ] Cotton pads
- [ ] Hand mirror

TOUCH-UP TIPS

Use your express makeup kit to touch up your makeup—fast. Here are some quick tips.

Skin

- If your skin is too shiny, use non-powdered blotting papers. They'll de-shine your skin in seconds and work better than powder.

- Tone down flushed skin with an anti-red primer. These are available at your cosmetic or pharmacy counter.

- In hot weather, which makes you perspire, use a grease-based foundation, as it's water-resistant and won't run.

- However, if your foundation is dripping, cool your face down first. Drink some cold water, wet a towel and throw it in the freezer for a minute, then drape it around your neck to cool down your body. Alternatively, wrap a few ice cubes in a clean table napkin and tie it around your neck. Another tip is to keep a cheap battery-operated face fan in your bag. It's safe, light and compact.

Eyes

- If you're always in a rush, consider keeping your eyebrows and lashes tinted to your desired colour, and invest in lash extensions so you don't need to apply mascara. They look incredibly natural and can last for up to six weeks. Waterproof mascara also helps.

- If your mascara runs, dab a small amount of foundation onto the end of a cotton bud and use it as an eraser.

- If your curled lashes are starting to straighten out like fence posts, warm up a heated eyelash curler and redo them.

- Before using a cotton bud to touch up around your eyes, especially the inner rims, wet it with eye drops. You'll not only soothe your eyes but also reduce the risk of leaving behind any fibres.

Lips

- Apply lip balm heavily to dry lips before you even start your makeup, then let it soak in. By the time you apply lipstick, you'll have luscious, soft lips that will make your lipstick easier to apply. It'll last longer too. I love using lip balm on cuticles, cracked heels and dry elbows.

- Bleeding lipstick? Wipe the whole lot off with a baby wipe and start again. But the real trick is to buy the most intense colours and only apply lipstick once—the less product on your lips, the less it will run. As I always say, too much on your mouth goes south.

- If your lip shape is 'responding' to gravity, don't draw attention to it by applying a bright shade of lipstick. Try this simple test. Apply your brightest lipstick, then look in the mirror, squinting your eyes until your vision is blurred. If your lip shape is plump and youthful, go for your life! If it looks aged or slightly droopy, choose a nude lip colour, which will give the illusion of fuller lips by making your lip borders less defined. If you want to add more colour to your face, apply more blush and mascara.

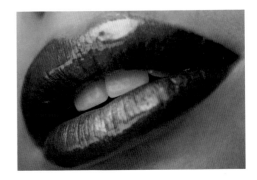

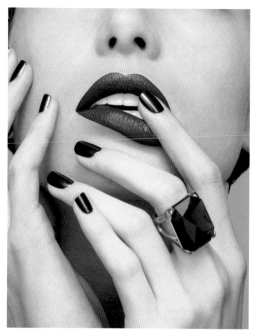

MODEL CASSI COLVIN – CHIC MANAGEMENT

After 5

If you're getting dressed up for a special night out, then you're probably adding bling to your ears, décolletage and hands. In other words, you're highlighting potential problem areas, which, depending on your age, may make you look years older.

- If your earlobes have become saggy from wearing heavy earrings, wear something a bit discreet and delicate.

- And if you can't resist wearing a plunging neckline but your décolletage concerns you, blend your makeup down to your dress rather than stop at your jawline. Use mineral foundation to cover this area, as it has a flawless finish as well as the best staying power; it is also less likely to appear on your clothes. Alternatively, simply wear a scarf.

Hands

- If you have red hands, resist the temptation to wear red nail polish—it has exactly the same effect as adding a red lipstick to red skin! Instead, always wear understated, skin-toned, non-shimmery polishes.

- Apply foundation to the backs of your hands to even out their skin tone and make them look years younger, then use a baby wipe to clean any foundation from your palms.

- For chipped, unmanicured nails, buy a nail buffer and use it to shine your natural nails. Believe me, you'll have the same shine as if you've used a clear nail polish.

Hair

- For greasy hair, use dry shampoo, which looks like deodorant in a can. It transforms greasy hair in seconds.

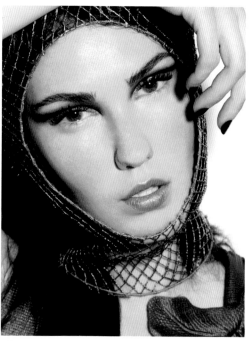

MODEL RACHAEL GRASSO – VIVIEN'S MODEL MANAGEMENT

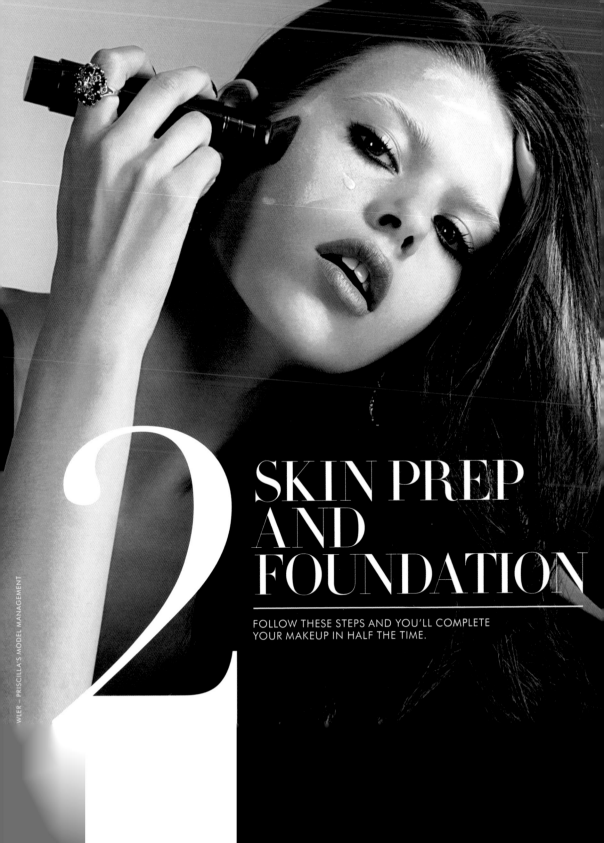

2

SKIN PREP AND FOUNDATION

FOLLOW THESE STEPS AND YOU'LL COMPLETE
YOUR MAKEUP IN HALF THE TIME.

THE EXPRESS PREP

There are two ways to prep your skin. The first way is obvious—prep your whole face by cleansing, moisturising and the weekly scrub. But there is an 'express' prep you can do when you've had makeup on all day and you just need to freshen up.

You don't have to start all over again and do the works. You can simply refresh your whole look by prepping your eyes. Not only will you apply makeup faster, but also your eye shadow will look more vibrant and last longer.

It's impossible to blend eye shadow on a very oily lid surface. Generally your eyelids are as oily, if not oilier, than your T-zone, and this is why eye shadow creases. (Your T-zone includes your centre forehead, the corners of your nostrils, the tip of your nose, your top lip and the middle of your chin.)

When I do makeup, whether the model is 15 or 50, I remove all the oil from the eyelids first. The eye makeup will then last for 6 to 8 hours without me having to retouch.

SKIN PREP ROUTINE

Follow these steps to start your makeup from scratch after work or before a night out but, if you don't have time to take everything off and start again, just refresh your eyes.

1 Cleanse

If you're nowhere near running water, use a non-alcoholic, non-perfumed baby wipe on your face and eyelids—a great tip if you're at the office and about to go out. It will remove all the oil, leaving no residue behind, so you can apply makeup straight on top. (All the others leave behind an oily residue that must be rinsed off; also, they can irritate your skin.)

2 Prime / moisturise

Makeup primer and moisturiser are essentially the same thing, except that a primer has more silicon, great for levelling out an uneven skin texture. I use either primer *or* moisturiser under foundation, as foundation needs to go into the skin and look like skin. Using more than one product underneath foundation makes it separate and look *patchy*, and it just doesn't last as long. So don't use both, and make sure that the one you choose contains a sunscreen.

It's important to ensure that your foundation, concealer, primer, sunscreen and moisturiser are all either oil-based or water-based. If you mix them, they'll separate.

3 Apply foundation and concealer

Don't moisturise your eyelids. Instead, put a light amount of foundation on your eyelids and/or concealer under your eyes. All foundations contain some form of moisture anyway, so you'll be doubling up in an area that just doesn't need it.

If you tend to have dark areas under your eyes, you may find your foundation is sufficient. But if it isn't, apply a little concealer over your foundation, and let your eye makeup begin.

Now read on and learn how to use foundation to create luminous, flawless skin that matches your skin tone perfectly.

FOUNDATION

There are so many foundations available today that I want to make it very easy for you to purchase foundation next time you hit the makeup counter.

Your skin type

Before you decide on a foundation, put yourself in one of these two categories.

NORMAL/OILY/BLEMISHED

Before you apply any foundation, first prep your skin (see opposite). As your skin already has a generous supply of oil, use a water-based foundation. Only use water-based moisturiser or primer in areas that are not excessively oily. Never go for a matte foundation, as it's too different to your natural texture. Sure, your skin, especially your T-zone, may grease up during the day, but you can easily remove the sheen by using non-powdered blotting papers as often as you like. This also keeps your skin creamy, so you can constantly reapply concealer or foundation as required. Remember, once you apply powder to your face, you can never just refresh your foundation—you'll have to take everything off and start all over again.

If you really want to achieve a velvety or matte skin, always blot before you powder, and remember that halfway through the day you may need to remove your whole foundation and start again. You can apply a good foundation in less than three minutes and leave your eye makeup intact.

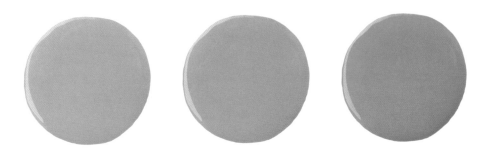

NORMAL/DRY

Normal to dry skin is a dream for long-lasting foundation. Just exfoliate your face once a week with this magical bicarb and cleanser mix, recommended by many dermatologists as a gentle and non-reactant exfoliant—simply combine a bit of warm water with half a teaspoon each of bicarbonate of soda and any good-quality water-based cleanser.

Always use a primer *or* moisturiser, and go for creamier, oil-based foundation. Your skin will drink it up like a sponge. And if you want a matte finish, go for it. Even if your skin feels dry, you may tend to get a bit of shine around the nose or forehead. Simply blot your T-zone with non-powdered blotting papers before you apply any powder.

Skin texture

When you choose foundation, base your decision on the skin 'texture' you want. Look at the list of foundation textures below and decide on the end result you want. Try experimenting—you might like to mix an eye look with one of the following foundation textures.

FOUNDATION TEXTURES

Here's a list of the different foundation textures, all of which are included in this book.

- **Sheer:**   Minimal coverage and an invisible finish.
- **Soft dewy/creamy:** Light to medium coverage.
- **Glowing/luminous:** Creamy, with extra shine/glow.
- **Velvety finish:**   Bare skin or foundation powdered with very sheer translucent powder.
- **Heavy coverage:**   Creamy, dewy finish (great for covering scars and blemishes).
- **Heavy coverage:**   Matte finish.

Your perfect colour match

There's one basic rule for choosing the right colour of foundation—match your foundation to the colour of your collarbone/décolletage (chest area). It's essential that your face and body are the same colour. If your skin tans, changing tone from summer to winter, always choose a matching foundation! I believe every woman should own a minimum of two shades.

Try the following exercise. Put on a singlet top and apply the foundation you currently use. Turn side on to the mirror and put your chin onto your shoulder. Your forehead should be the same colour as your chin, shoulder, arm, knee, even right down to your ankle. Think of two extreme skin tones—say, Anne Hathaway's versus Beyoncé's. Their foreheads match their chests, their shoulders, their knees, their elbows.

Never match your foundation to your jawline, as your neck area is one of the palest parts of your body.

Only use tinted sunscreens on blemish-free skin, as they don't provide good coverage.

Applying foundation

To apply foundation, always use your hands or a foundation brush (my fibre-optic brush is my favourite). I *never* use a sponge. It may seem like a cheap alternative, but it's expensive in the long run because more foundation is absorbed by the sponge than by your skin. And if you don't wash it after *every* use, it will be full of bacteria.

Natural daylight is best for applying makeup; never leave the house without checking your makeup in the best natural light. And if you're doing your makeup at night, make sure your globe is the type that replicates natural daylight. The best place for checking daytime makeup is in the rear-view mirror of a car, because it reflects so much natural light back onto your face. It's also a great way to pick up those few stray lip or eyebrow hairs.

Powder

Never powder your base just to make your makeup last longer. Yes, powder your bare skin if you want the finished look to be velvety/less shiny or matte, but never powder your base. Let's say, for example, that your non-powdered foundation lasts perfectly on your skin for three hours before it starts to slightly separate and deteriorate. As a result, you decide to pick up some powder and apply it, hoping for an all-day lasting effect (which is impossible). When you do this, you change your desired youthful dewy skin to powdered matte skin that may look caked and heavy.

The second you powder your skin, you can never go back and reapply your cream concealer or liquid foundation to touch up—you can only reapply more powder.

Anti-shine primer

If you're a shiner, buy a packet of either non-powdered blotting papers or some anti-shine primer or cream, which makes excess oil evaporate. Your skin will look instantly matte. Use it only on oily skin or your T-zone, for obvious reasons. Apply it with either a sponge or a foundation brush. If you can't find this anti-shine product in the department stores, call a professional makeup supplier in your area.

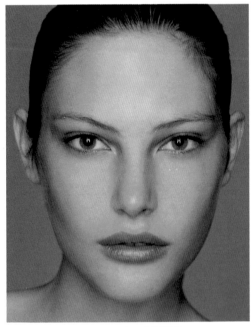

Anti-shine primer is mainly used on male actors who tend to get overly shiny and don't want to wear even a hint of makeup. It's also amazing on bald men whose heads shine like light bulbs.

MODEL CATHERINE MCNEIL – CHIC MANAGEMENT

11

Mineral foundations

I love mineral foundations, as they're great on sensitive skins and most of them have sunscreens. Powdered mineral foundations need to be polished into the skin with a brush, not lightly dusted over it. Women who love the mineral revolution tend to go heavy on the oily moisturisers prior to application, but by the time mineral foundation hits moisturised oily skin, it sticks like glue. So only lightly moisturise your skin, then let it become completely absorbed before you apply mineral foundation.

Only choose the powdered version if you desire a velvety matte finish. For a dewy, creamy effect, choose the liquid one.

Luminisers

One of the most fabulous tricks of the trade, these pots of golden creamy sheen come in at least three shades, suitable for pale, medium and black skins. Giving your skin an incredible glow is so easy to achieve—simply add a couple of drops to your foundation.

Highlighters

When you only want to shimmer up certain areas of your face, see 'Highlighting', opposite, as well as my easy step-by-step instructions on pages 15–16.

CONCEALING BLEMISHES

If blemishes are ruining your life, consult a dermatologist. Always buy densely pigmented concealers, as you can always blend them down. Here's a trick for testing a concealer at the makeup counter—first use a red felt pen to draw a tiny red circle on the back of your hand, then try different concealers until you find one that can cover that red spot completely and still leave your skin looking natural.

Applying concealer

Any makeup that is lighter than your skin's natural shade will highlight and raise indentations, while any makeup that is darker than your skin's natural shade will flatten. If you're covering a scar or deep, dark circles under your eyes, or anything that sits below the skin's surface, such as a hole or dint, choose a concealer that's one to two shades paler than your foundation.

On the other hand, if you're concealing a blemish or a mole or a raised imperfection (in other words, something that's above the skin's surface), you need to choose a concealer that is the exact shade of your foundation, maybe even half a shade darker, so that it will both flatten and minimise. Using a light concealer on a raised blemish will actually highlight it!

HIGHLIGHTING

You can highlight your skin by mixing a liquid highlighter (a luminiser) with foundation and applying it all over your face—fabulous for young and blemish-free skin—or you can highlight only certain features, giving your skin a hint of a glow while avoiding problem areas.

The best tip for choosing the right highlighter colour is to first apply the product to the cupid's bow on your top lip. You should see a natural shine, as if your natural skin tone is glowing, not colour. If it's too yellow, you've chosen a colour that's too dark for your skin tone. If it looks white and frosty, you've chosen a colour that's too light.

For example, look at the pigments below, which are all categorised according to skin tone.

For paler skin tones, use really sheer 'eggshell' soft gold pigments or creams.

For medium skin tones, use soft golds and rose golds, not bronzes.

For dark skins, use deep golds and bronzes like these.

For black skins, use burgundies and dark, shimmery chocolate.

Where to highlight

If you want to achieve a luminous, beautiful look, follow these rules for highlighting your skin.

- For youthful, wrinkle-free skin, you can luminise all over. Just add a few drops of luminising liquid to your base.
- If you're even slightly worried about fine lines and blemishes, follow the step-by-step technique on pages 15–16. You can choose to highlight all the areas shown on page 14, or only a few.
- Don't use highlighter on areas where your skin is extremely oily, blemished or lined.
- Highlight the inner corners of your eyes, which rarely wrinkle as you age, to bring light into your eyes and perk them up if they're tired. Choose a highlighter that matches your skin tone.

FOREHEAD

UPPER
CHEEK
BONE

NOSE
BRIDGE

CUPID'S
BOW

INNER EYE
CORNER

MIDDLE
EYELID

BROW
BONE

Highlighting tips

- Only use white or silver greys for highlighting the inner corners of your eyes.
- Make sure your cupid's bow is hair-free—girls, we don't highlight our lip hair!
- Avoid highlighters that reflect purple tones—always check your product on the back of your hand to make sure there are no purple/pink reflections.
- If your brow is slightly hooded, don't draw attention to this area by highlighting it.
- Don't use cream highlighter on your eyelids—creams crease and eyelids move, so they're not a good combination. But creams are fabulous everywhere else, especially on your cheekbones.
- Never use a frosty white eye shadow, and never, ever highlight your whole brow bone.

1 EYELIDS

To avoid fallout, first wet an angle brush. Apply highlighter to the inner corners of your eyes, then look down and apply it to the centre of your eyelids.

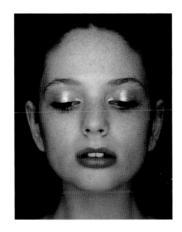

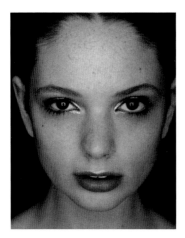

2 CUPID'S BOW

Using the same wet brush, highlight your top lip, the cupid's bow. You can see how this instantly makes your lips fuller, and you don't have to obviously overdraw your lip line.

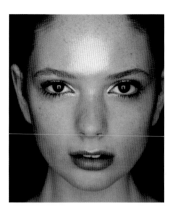

3 NOSE

Highlight down the centre of your nose, but be careful not to go to the very tip. (If you're over-oily in this area, don't highlight your nose at all.)

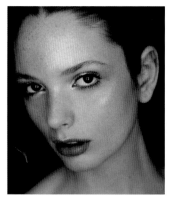

4 FOREHEAD

With a kabuki brush, apply highlighter to the centre of your forehead. This gives the very youthful illusion of a rounded forehead, and is great for normal to dry skin. Again, avoid this area if it is oily.

5 CHEEKS & BROWS

Using your fingertip or a fan brush, apply a hint of highlighter to your cheekbone. You should only be able to see this highlight when you turn side on. If you can see it front on, you've used too much. Avoid this area if you're heavily lined. Wetting a fine angle brush, highlight very closely along the last third of your eyebrow. Keep this section very thin so you don't create a puffy eyelid. Highlighting the whole brow bone creates an ageing effect.

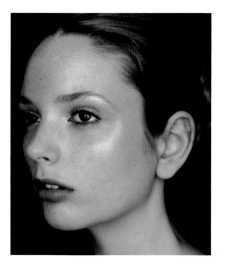

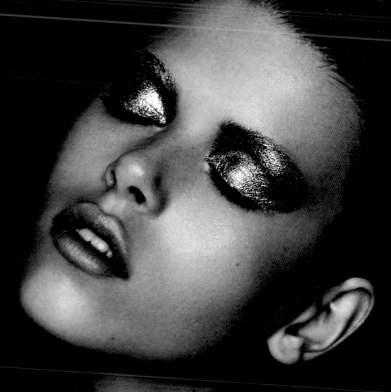

3 EYES

TRANSFORM YOUR
LOOK WITH THE BEST
ACCESSORY YOU'LL
EVER OWN.

LASHES

Nothing can change or enhance an eye as quickly as a false lash. As this is an express makeup book, I'm only going to talk about false eyelashes that are quick and easy to apply (these might be hard to find, so look up my faves on www.raemorris.com). If you are buying them elsewhere, remember to check that they're an exact fit, because they completely change both your eye shape and the overall look of your makeup.

Always apply lashes with waterproof latex so, if you cry, the lashes won't fall off. Most lashes come with a small complimentary tube, but it's great if you can track down one that's made with duo latex, which can be found in every makeup artist's kit. I've also discovered a magic tool, known as an eyelash applicator (also available on my website).

Always check the base of the lash, which will be either clear or black. This is the seam to which all the lashes are sown. If the seam is black, you will get an eyeliner effect on your eyelids. If it's clear, the false lashes will look more natural, blending in with your own lashes without giving that eyeliner effect.

As you browse through the following steps, you'll be able to see the difference between clear- and black-seamed lashes. You'll also see how powerful false eyelashes can be. I've just curled the model's natural lashes and applied a fine, soft wash of mascara.

To remove lashes, hold a cotton bud dipped in warm water over your eye for about two minutes. The latex should fall away easily.

Don't apply false lashes the whole length of your lash line, as they will drag down your eye. Always move them in a millimetre or two from the outer edge.

Natural

In this shot our model is wearing only a little mascara on her natural lashes, and no other eye makeup. As you look at the following shots, compare them to this look to see what you can achieve with different lashes.

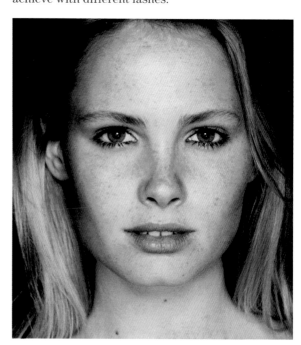

MODEL SHANAY HALL –
VIVIEN'S MODEL MANAGEMENT

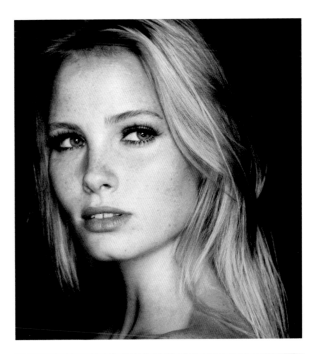

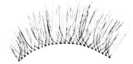

Wispy lash

The first lash I've used is quite soft, and wispy on the ends. It has a clear lash line, giving a natural look. I like to use it on women who have never worn false eyelashes before. They're easy to apply and look fabulous.

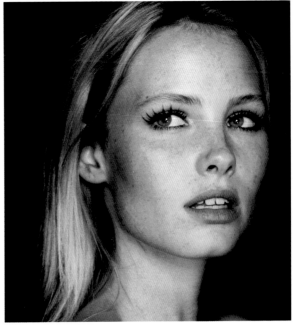

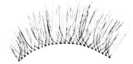

Separated lash

Similar to the 3/4 lash (see page 20) and easy to apply, the separated lash is great if you want your top lash to look more defined. Again, the base is clear, so it doesn't give you a heavy eyeliner effect.

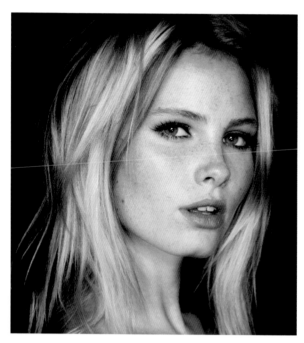

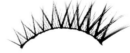

3/4 lash

This 3/4 lash is the type I use most, as it fits every eyelid and is easy to apply. The base is black, so it will give you an eyeliner effect. However, as the lash only goes three-quarters of the way across your eyelid, you'll have to extend your eyeliner. I have smudged some black kohl pencil onto an angled brush and extended the line into the inner corner of each eye, as shown.

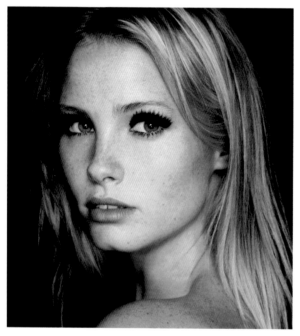

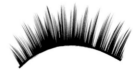

Full lash

This is one of the fullest lashes you can use—any fuller and you'll look like a drag queen. Before you apply it, check the length of the false lash against your natural eyelash line. If they differ in length, you may want to trim half a centimetre from the end of each lash before applying them.

BROWS

Over-arching your eyebrow creates a puffy eyelid that instantly ages you about ten years and adds 5 kilos (or more) to your face! Remember—when you straighten your brow and lower the arch, you create a younger, more sophisticated look. Here are the three worst brow crimes you can commit.

If you have stray grey brow hairs, be sure to match the colour of your brows to your natural hair colour.

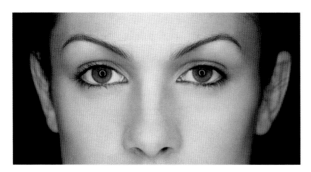

The triangle

As you can see, a triangular-shaped brow gives you a natural frown that says 'I'm annoyed' without even trying. Never angle your eyebrows to this extreme. By lifting the brow at the dead centre of each eye, the downhill slant you create at the end of your brows is not only ageing but also creates a huge, saggy, puffy eyelid.

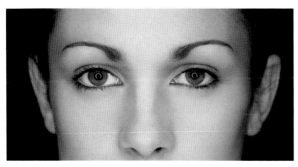

The tadpole

The tadpole brow creates a hard, angry, severe effect that looks 1980s and 1920s at the same time, but in an unflattering way—the further apart your brows are, the wider your nose looks. This shape starts with a thick Brooke Shields brow, then suddenly changes into a thin pencil line.

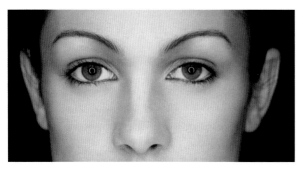

The letter 'M'

This unflattering shape creates—yet again—unattractive puffy, droopy eyes and also adds years to your face. It's also the worst shape if you have saggy, heavy lids. Only use it if you have a very flat eyelid, or if you're addicted to the 'flapper' look from the 1920s and wear the polished, perfectly groomed makeup to match.

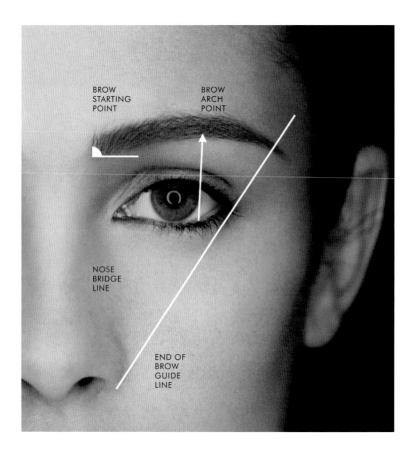

BROW
STARTING
POINT

BROW
ARCH
POINT

NOSE
BRIDGE
LINE

END OF
BROW
GUIDE
LINE

The perfect brow

With an arch that cuts through the brow bone, the perfect brow straightens and narrows your nose and lifts your eyes. The less you arch your brows, the younger you'll look.

Nose bridge line Here's the rule—set the gap between your brows to match your desired nose bridge width, and you'll create the illusion of a thinner, more refined nose.

Brow starting point Make sure this is at a right angle. Keeping the bottom hairs on a perfect horizontal line will lift your eyes. You may have to pluck any stray hairs under it.

Brow arch point The point where you should lift your brow is two-thirds of the way across your brow, in line with the outer edge of your iris. If you have stray hairs between your brow and your hairline, pluck away.

End of brow guide line Imagine a line from the corner of your nose to the outer corner of your eye and out, then make sure your brows don't fall short of it, otherwise your eyes will look distorted and your brows will give you a severe, masculine expression.

4

EYE COLOUR CHARTS

YOUR EYES ARE NOT ONLY THE
WINDOWS TO YOUR SOUL BUT ALSO
THE FIRST THING PEOPLE NOTICE.

FINDING THE RIGHT COLOUR

One of the best things you can do for your makeup is enhance your eyes. Even if you perfectly colour match your outfit to your complexion, the wrong eye shadow can bring it all undone. Sometimes even I get confused about the difference between someone having a 'warm/cool' or 'summer/winter' skin tone, as it's based on a combination of your skin, eyes and hair, and the three are not always the same tone. (You can have warm eyes with cool skin, or warm skin with cool hair.)

On the following pages, the natural eye colours have been grouped into both warm and cool. Simply locate your eye colour in the centre of one of the colour charts, and you'll find the perfect eye shadow colours for you. The eye shadow charts are also divided into two groups— colours that complement your natural eye colour, and colours that intensify it, making it pop.

The chart below suits all eye colours, so I recommend you have two or three of these eye shadow colours in your makeup kit.

All the shades we've chosen can also be used as eyeliners, pencils or highlighters, which come in either a matte or metallic finish.

ALL EYE COLOURS

Neutral colours

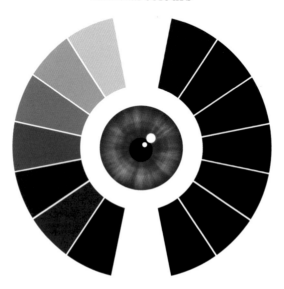

BLUE EYES

Warm blue

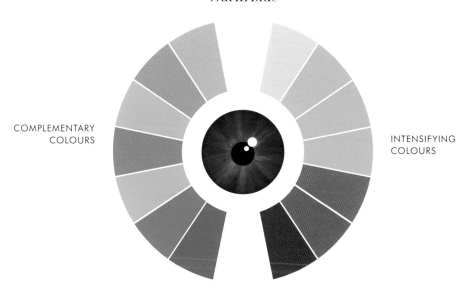

COMPLEMENTARY
COLOURS

INTENSIFYING
COLOURS

Cool blue

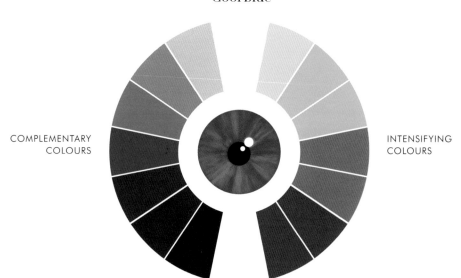

COMPLEMENTARY
COLOURS

INTENSIFYING
COLOURS

BROWN EYES

Warm brown

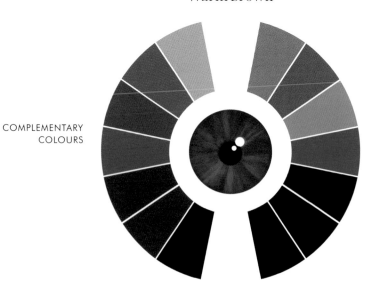

COMPLEMENTARY
COLOURS

INTENSIFYING
COLOURS

Cool brown

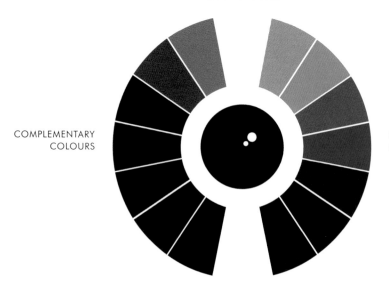

COMPLEMENTARY
COLOURS

INTENSIFYING
COLOURS

GREEN EYES

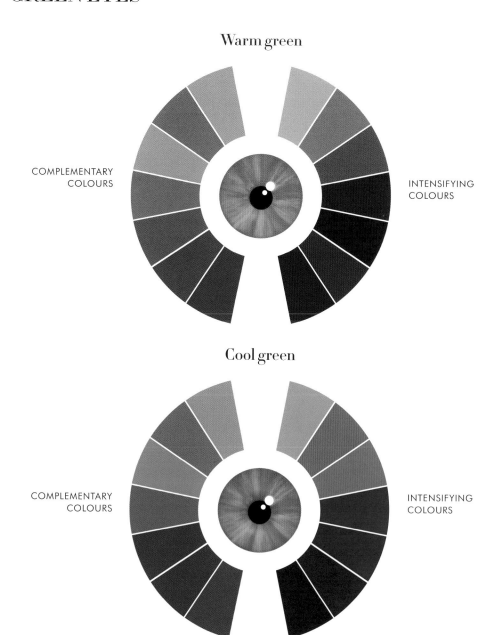

Warm green

COMPLEMENTARY
COLOURS

INTENSIFYING
COLOURS

Cool green

COMPLEMENTARY
COLOURS

INTENSIFYING
COLOURS

HAZEL EYES

True hazel

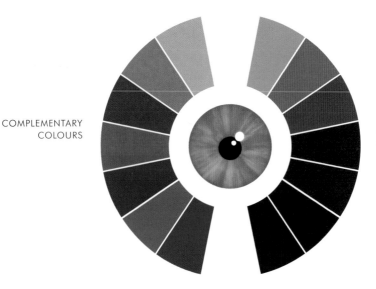

COMPLEMENTARY
COLOURS

INTENSIFYING
COLOURS

Golden hazel

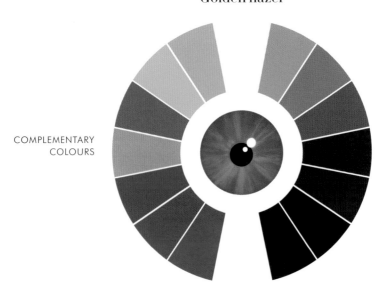

COMPLEMENTARY
COLOURS

INTENSIFYING
COLOURS

5

EXPRESS LOOKS

HERE ARE LOTS OF KILLER LOOKS
THAT YOU CAN PULL OFF FAST.

1 | NATURAL GLAMOUR

A CLEAR VERSATILE
LOOK THAT SUITS
ALL SKIN TONES.

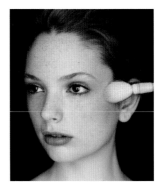

1 | PREP & FOUNDATION

Prep your skin, then apply light foundation and concealer. For a velvety finish, add light translucent powder. Finish by applying a mineral powdered blush with a kabuki brush.

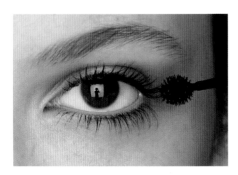

2 | LASHES

Curl your eyelashes, then apply lots of black mascara to your top and bottom lashes.

3 | LIPS

Apply a red lipstick that suits your skin tone. For example, orange-reds make your teeth look yellow but burgundy-reds make your teeth look whiter.

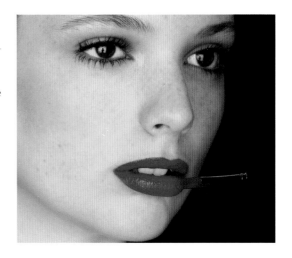

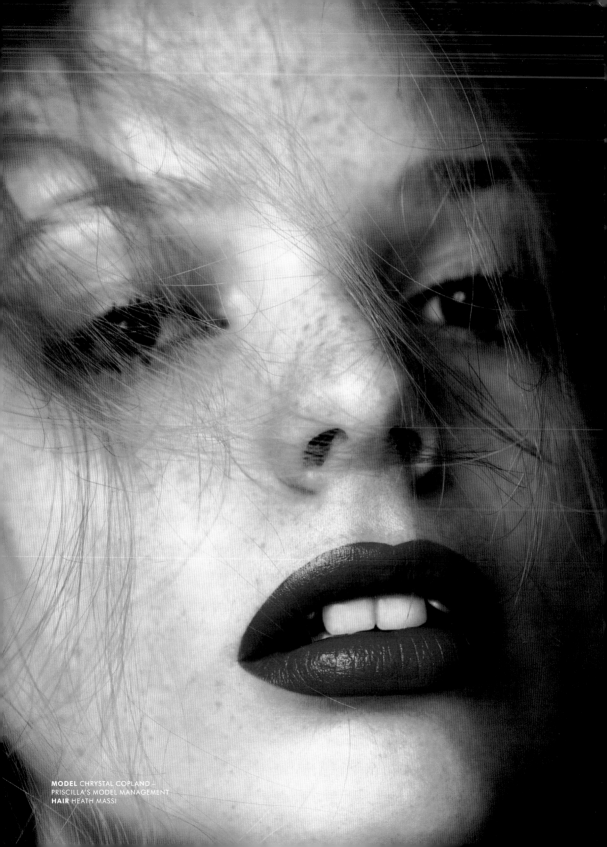

MODEL CHRYSTAL COPLAND –
PRISCILLA'S MODEL MANAGEMENT
HAIR HEATH MASSI

2 | AUBERGINE VELVET

RICH VIOLET WITH THE
DEFINITION YOU GET
FROM A SMOKY EYE.

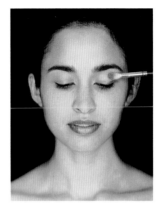

1 EYE PREP & FOUNDATION

Prep your skin,
making sure you
remove all the oil
from your eyelids.
Apply foundation
to your eyelids, then
lightly powder them.

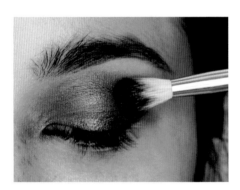

2 EYE SHADOW

Now apply a rich violet pigment to
each eyelid, blending to just under
the brow bone. Ignore the messy
fallout, which you can clean up
later. To intensify the colour, wet
your brush.

3 UPPER DEFINITION & BLENDING

Use black eye shadow or
gel eyeliner to blend the
socket line. For better
blending, apply gentle
pressure and extend the
line outwards as shown.

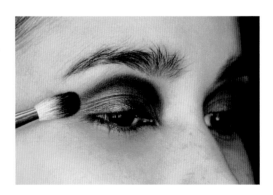

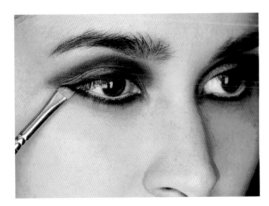

4 LOWER DEFINITION & BLENDING

With a fine angle brush, apply black gel eyeliner along the lower and upper lash lines, and softly blend. Then use a creamy white pencil to line inside your inner eyelids.

5 FINISHING EYES & FOUNDATION

Use a baby wipe to clean up any eye shadow fallout from under your eyes, then apply foundation mixed with a luminiser. Define your eyebrows. Curl your lashes and apply lots of black mascara. Finally, apply a cream coral blush to your cheeks.

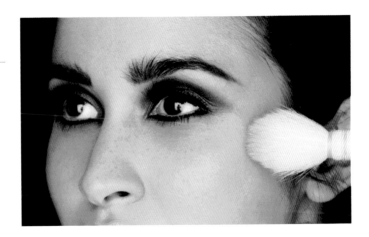

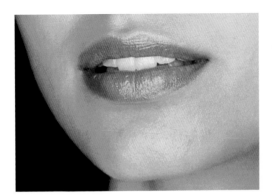

6 LIPS

Finish with a matching coral lipstick.

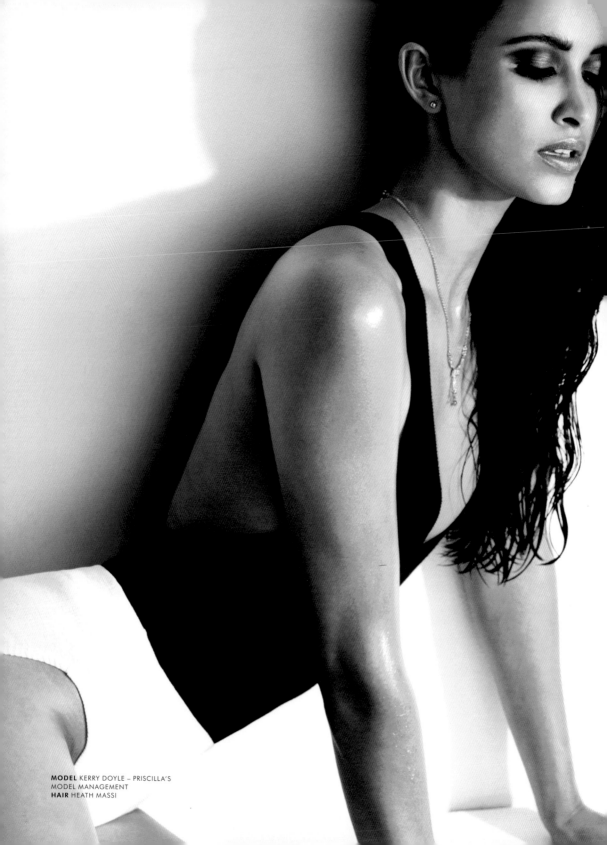

MODEL KERRY DOYLE – PRISCILLA'S
MODEL MANAGEMENT
HAIR HEATH MASSI

3 COCO DESIRE

HERE'S THE QUICK
WAY TO APPLY THE
CLASSIC CAT EYE.

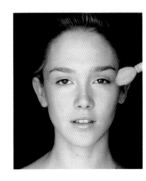

1 FOUNDATION & BLUSH

Define your brows, and
apply sheer foundation
before lightly powdering
your entire face. Apply a
soft beige blush to your
cheeks, and a wash of
blush over your eyelids.

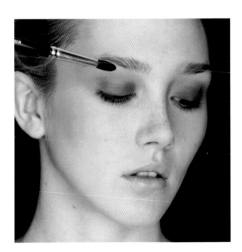

2 EYE SHADOW

Using an eye shadow brush, do a
soft wash of a matte taupe—think
matte brown—eye shadow around
your entire eye. Repeat for the other
eye. Do most of this looking straight
ahead, as you want this colour to
just lightly creep up under your
brow bone.

To help you blend, keep a clean
brush with translucent powder
on standby. When smudging kohl
pencil on your eyelids, turn the
brush upside down. This keeps the
intensity along the lash lines,
giving you a stronger effect.

3 UPPER & LOWER DEFINITION

Using a chocolate-brown pencil, smudge around the entire lash line, top and bottom, then blend with the mini square blending brush. Repeat for the other eye.

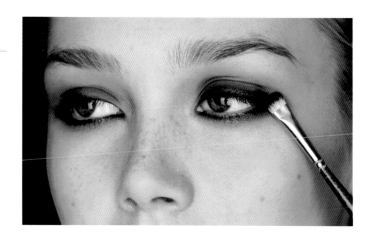

4 LASHES, BROWS & LIPS

Curl your lashes, and apply lots of black mascara to the top lashes only, then apply false wispy lashes. This will give you more of a cat-eye effect. Finish the look with a nude lipstick and, finally, add a defined, filled-in brow.

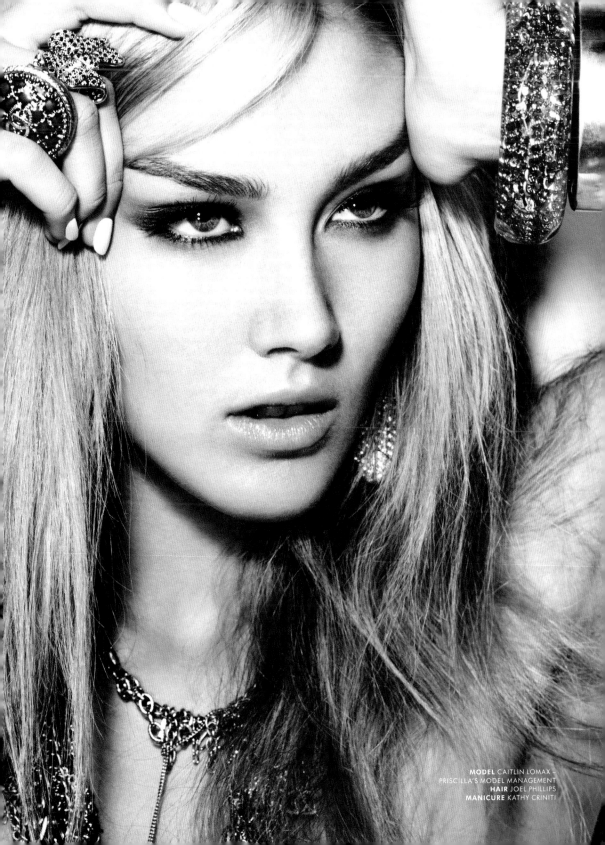

MODEL CAITLIN LOMAX –
PRISCILLA'S MODEL MANAGEMENT
HAIR JOEL PHILLIPS
MANICURE KATHY CRINITI

4 | SOFT CORAL

SOFT SHADES THAT SUIT ALL SKINS AND ALL AGES. A DIVINE DAY LOOK.

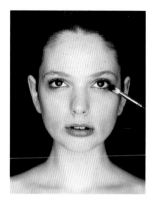

1 PREP & FOUNDATION

Prep your skin, then apply liquid foundation all over your face, powdering your eyelids only. Apply a soft pink blush to your eyelids and along your bottom lash lines.

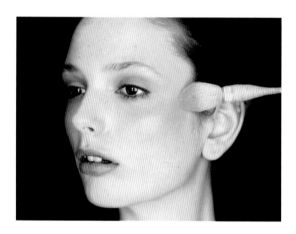

2 CHEEKS & LIPS

Use a kabuki brush to apply a cream coral blush to your cheeks and lips. This will give them a luminous texture.

3 LASHES

Curl your lashes, then apply mascara.

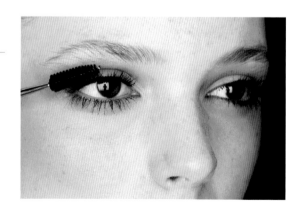

If your eyes are looking tired, apply creamy white pencil to the inner rims of each eye.

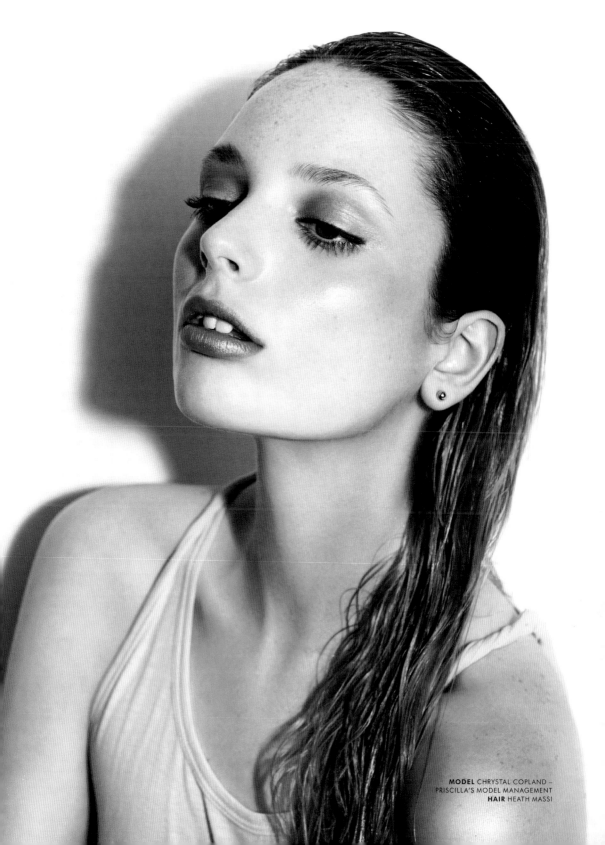

5 | LUSH BLUSH

A FEMININE, SULTRY EYE THAT ALL WOMEN DESIRE.

1 PREP & FOUNDATION

Apply foundation all over your face, then lightly powder all over, including your eyelids. Groom and define your eyebrows (see 'The perfect brow', page 22).

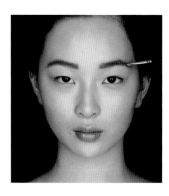

2 LOWER DEFINITION

Apply a chocolate-brown pencil to your outer bottom lash lines. Blend with a chocolate-brown eye shadow.

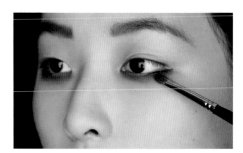

3 EYE SHADOW

Smudge pencil on your outer top lash lines. Look straight ahead and apply the same chocolate-brown eye shadow to your upper lids. Fill in the lids later. Blend at the edges with translucent powder.

Add a soft highlight to your nose and to the cupid's bow on your top lip (see 'Highlighting', pages 13–16).

4 LASHES, CHEEKS & LIPS

Curl your eyelashes, then apply mascara and false separated lashes. Use a kabuki brush to apply blush to your cheeks. Finish off with a soft apricot blush and lip balm on your lips.

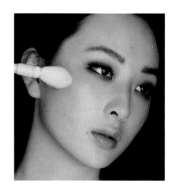

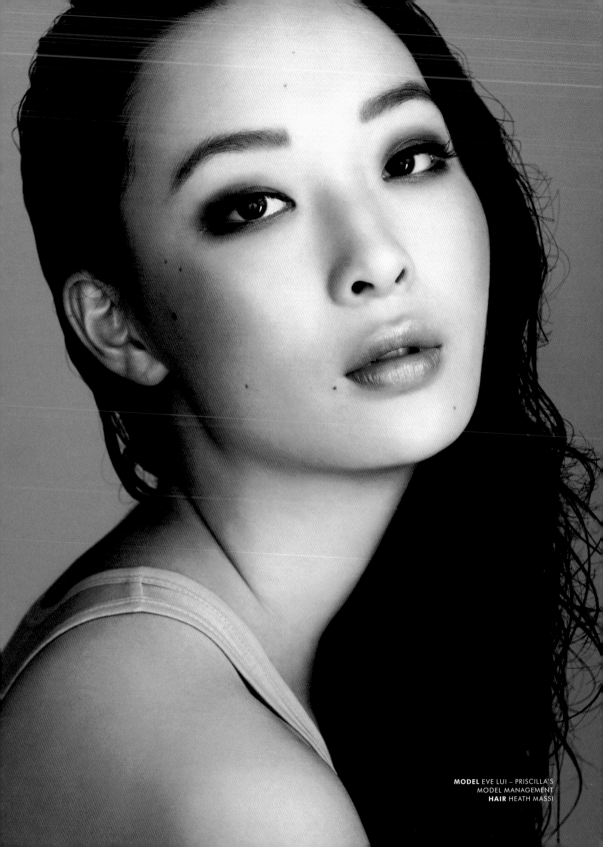

6 | PASTEL BOMB

CREAMY SKIN AND
PEACHY SHADES,
DAY OR NIGHT.

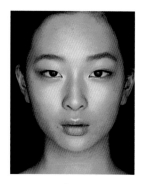

1 BRONZER & HIGHLIGHTER

This look requires bronzer, so I'm using a foundation four shades darker than the model's natural skin tone. Only do this if your body is tanned or dark/olive (the model had a spray tan). After bronzing, highlight your skin and groom your brows.

2 EYE SHADOW

While looking straight ahead, use a bright metallic orange eye shadow around the whole of each eye, then blend the outer edge with a soft coral pink.

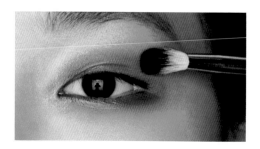

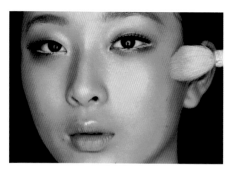

3 EYES & CHEEKS

Apply a creamy white pencil to the inner rim of each eye. After curling your lashes, add black mascara and false 3/4 lashes. Finally, apply metallic peach blush to each cheek. Eye shadow pigments are also great for this.

4 LIPS

Apply a soft, sheer baby-pink lip gloss.

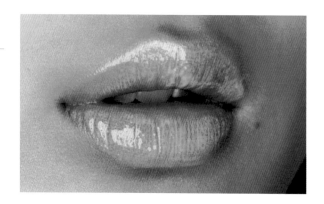

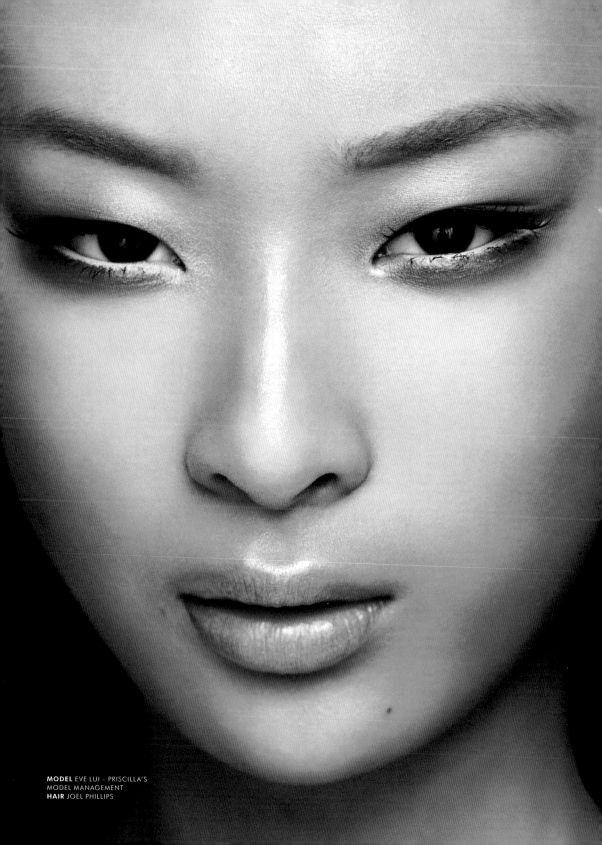

7 | EBONY RICH

A HOT BUT UTTERLY
TIMELESS LOOK FOR
ANY OCCASION.

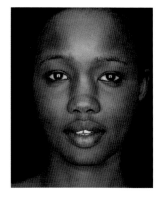

1 PREP, FOUNDATION & POWDER

Prep your skin. Apply foundation, and use a matte powder to kill any shine. I love it when black/dark skins are matte, as it softens the look.

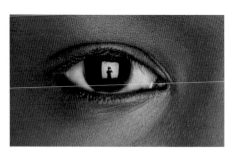

2 EYELINER & LASHES

To open up your eyes, apply a bone- or beige-coloured pencil to the inner rim of each eyelid. Apply an intense liquid black eyeliner along your top eyelids. Then curl your lashes, apply mascara and finish with false 3/4 lashes.

3 EYE SHADOW & BROWS

Use a black gel eyeliner as eye shadow. This is great for intense eyes and lasts all night. Just make sure you blend it quickly, as it dries fast. Then define your brows.

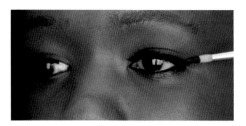

To define your eyes, apply a few extra coats of black gel eyeliner into both your eye sockets.

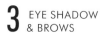

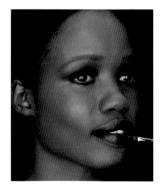

4 EYELINER & LIPS

Apply the same black gel eyeliner underneath the bottom lash line. Finish with a burgundy-black lipstick and a deep burgundy blush.

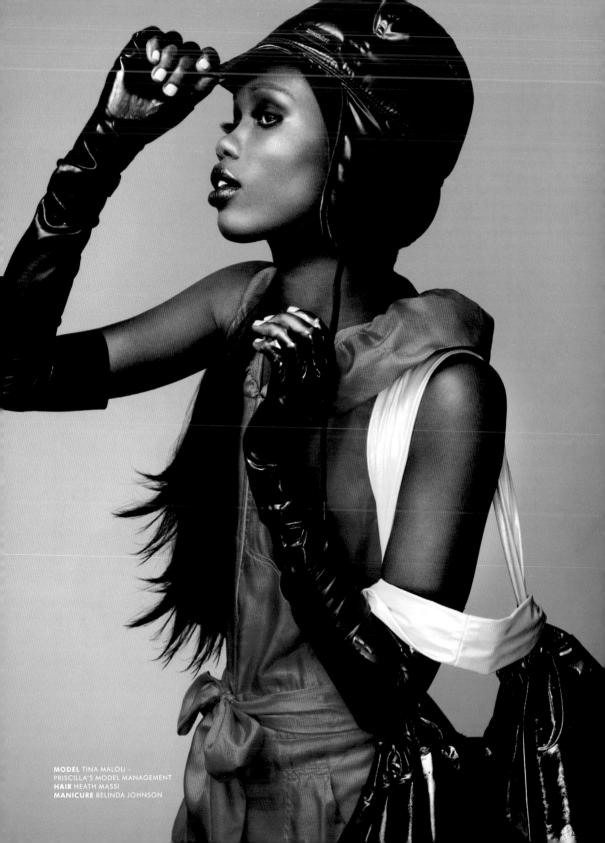

8 | ATOMIC ORANGE

LIVEN UP BROWN
SHADES WITH
INTENSE ORANGE.

1 EYE SHADOW

Prep your eyelids and
apply a shimmery bronze
eye shadow to your entire
lids. Don't worry about
any fallout, as you can
clean it up later. Use a
soft bronze eye shadow
to blend it up to each
brow bone, just under
your eyebrow.

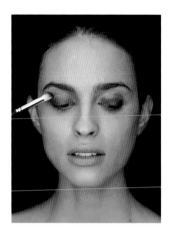

2 EYELINER

Wet a fine angle brush
and use it to apply an
intense orange pigment
as an eyeliner along each
top eyelash line.

*The best nudes are the colours
between your natural lip
colour and your natural skin
colour. If you use a lipstick
that's the same colour as
your foundation, you'll look
as if you have no lips.*

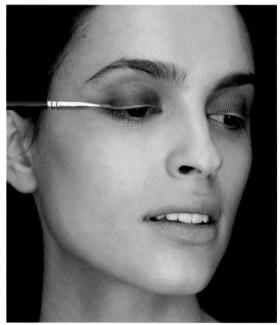

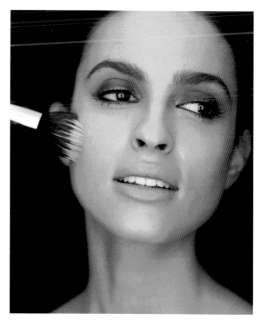

3 EYES, FOUNDATION & HIGHLIGHTER

Curl your lashes, and apply lots of mascara to both your top and bottom lashes. Apply a chocolate kohl eye pencil to the inner rim of each eye. Clean up any fallout and apply liquid foundation. Highlight your skin if you wish (see pages 13–16).

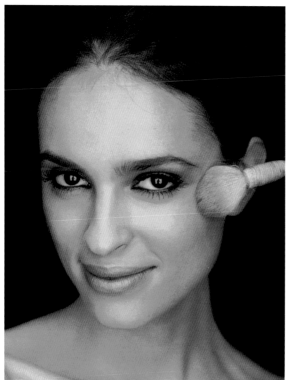

4 CHEEKS & LIPS

Apply a really soft cream burgundy blush to your cheeks, then use your finger to slightly stain your lip with the same blush. Next, apply a cream apricot blush to your cheeks. Finally, highlight your lips and apply a soft nude lipstick.

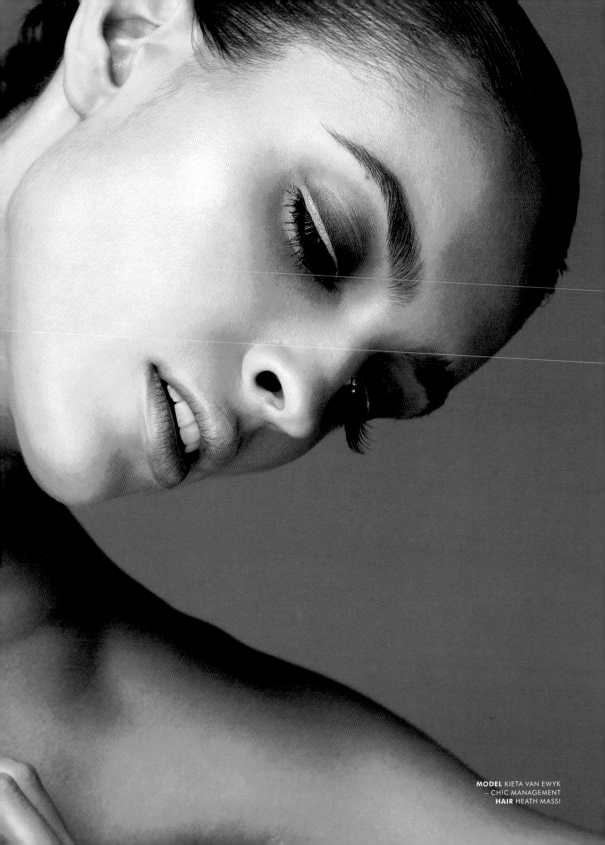

MODEL KIETA VAN EWYK
– CHIC MANAGEMENT
HAIR HEATH MASSI

9 | ULTRA LUX

A LUXURIOUS LOOK
FOR A GLAMOROUS
RED CARPET EVENT.

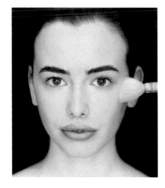

1 PREP, FOUNDATION & POWDER

Prep your skin, then apply foundation and concealer, and lightly powder your face. This will give your skin a velvety texture. Apply soft beige nude lipstick to your lips.

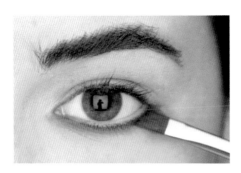

2 EYELINER

Smudge a reddish brown kohl pencil along your lash lines, then blend it with a clean brush.

3 UPPER DEFINITION & BLENDING

Colour in your whole eyelid with an intense black kohl pencil, then take a medium-sized brush and blend, blend, blend. Repeat for the other eye.

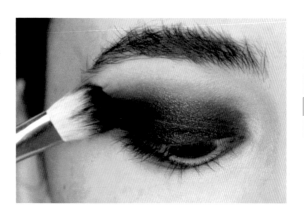

4 EYE SHADOW & BLENDING

Looking straight ahead, use a burgundy-red eye shadow to blend the black closer to your eyebrows.

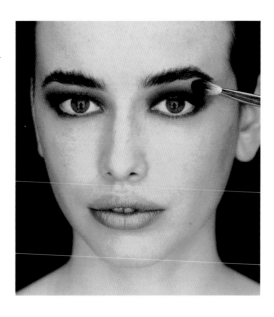

5 LASHES, CHEEKS & BROWS

Smudge more black kohl pencil into your bottom lash lines. Curl your lashes, then apply lots of mascara to your top and bottom lashes. Add false 3/4 lashes. Finish off with a soft peach blush and, finally, define your brows.

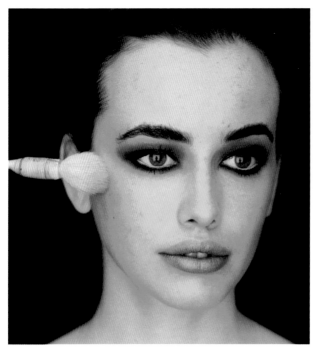

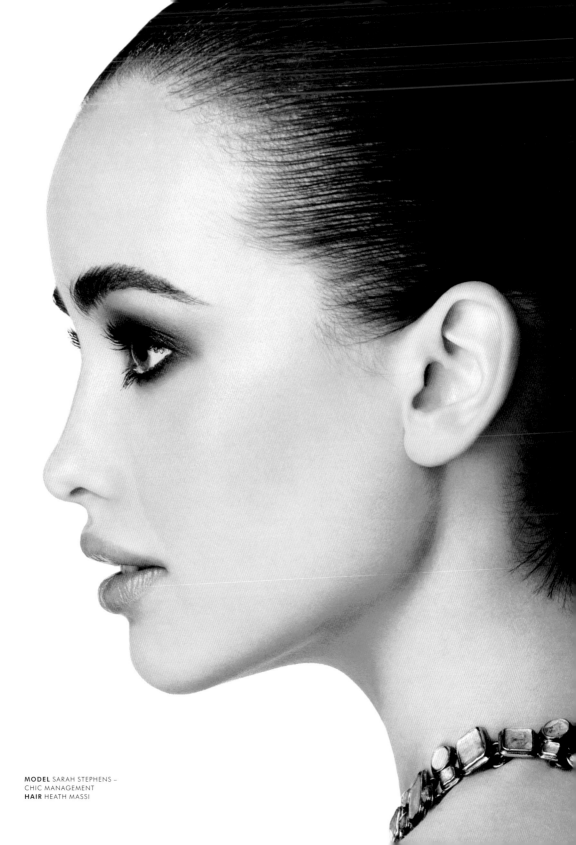

10

KOHL GLAMOUR

AN UNDERSTATED
SULTRY LOOK FOR
WOMEN OF ALL AGES.

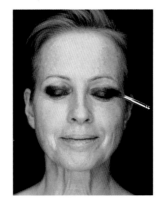

1 PREP & EYE SHADOW

Prep your skin, then lightly
powder your lids. Apply a
soft wash of matte brown
eye shadow, keeping the
intensity close to your
eyelash line. Then, using
an eye shadow brush,
smudge a kohl chocolate-
brown pencil along the top
of each eyelash line.

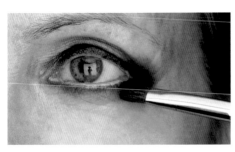

2 LOWER DEFINITION & BLENDING

Next, use a creamy white pencil on the inner rim
of each eye to help conceal redness and tiredness.
Apply a soft wash of matte brown eye shadow
under each eye, and blend well. Finally, apply a
chocolate-brown gel eyeliner, which is waterproof,
and softly blend under the eye.

3 LASHES, BROWS & FOUNDATION

Curl your lashes and apply lots of black mascara top and
bottom, then—if you're game—add some lashes. Clean
away any fallout, apply a liquid foundation and define
your brows. The model's eyebrows are naturally ash, so
to make them look more beautiful I put brown mascara
through them. When you fill in your brow, make sure you
match the pencil to your brow colour.

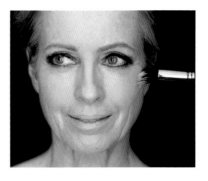

*Matte colours help disguise
wrinkles. It's important to do
90% of your makeup looking
straight ahead. If there's a
wrinkle or a crease, just put
colour straight over it.*

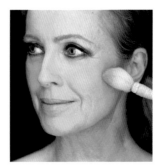

4 POWDER, CHEEKS & LIPS

Apply a soft translucent
powder all over your face,
then a soft peach blush
and matching lip colour.

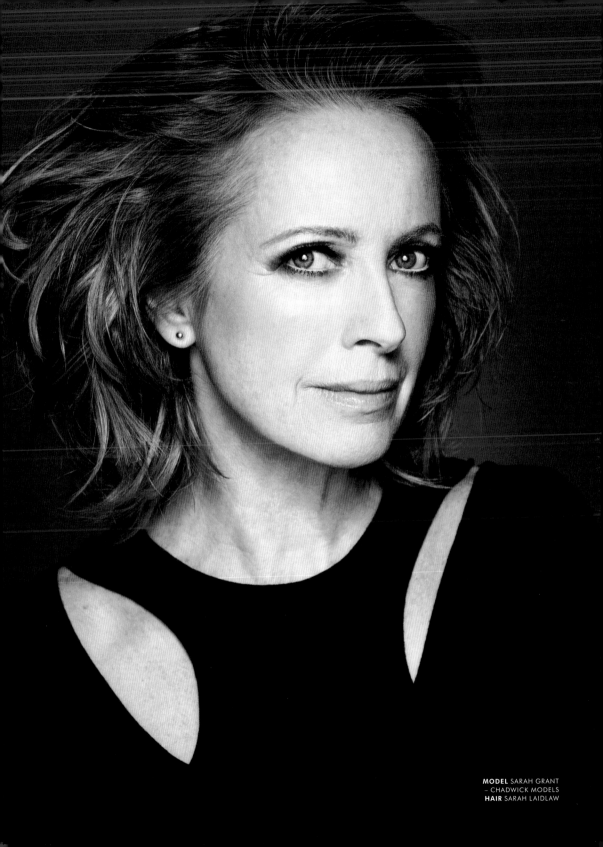

11 | NOIR CANDY

A PREPPY, FRESH LOOK THAT'S GREAT FOR ANY TIME, ANY PLACE.

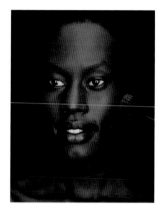

1 PREP, FOUNDATION & POWDER

Prep your skin, apply foundation and then apply a matte powder all over. Define your brows, and apply a deep matte burgundy blush to your cheeks (you can also use an eye shadow for this) and blend. Clean up any fallout.

2 EYES & LIPS

Curl your lashes, then apply mascara to your top and bottom lashes. Add false separated lashes. Run a black liquid eyeliner along the top and bottom of each eyelid. Finally, apply a deep burgundy lipstick.

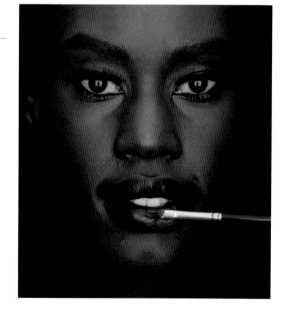

Because the model's brows are naturally so arched, I brought the arch down to give her a more sophisticated look.

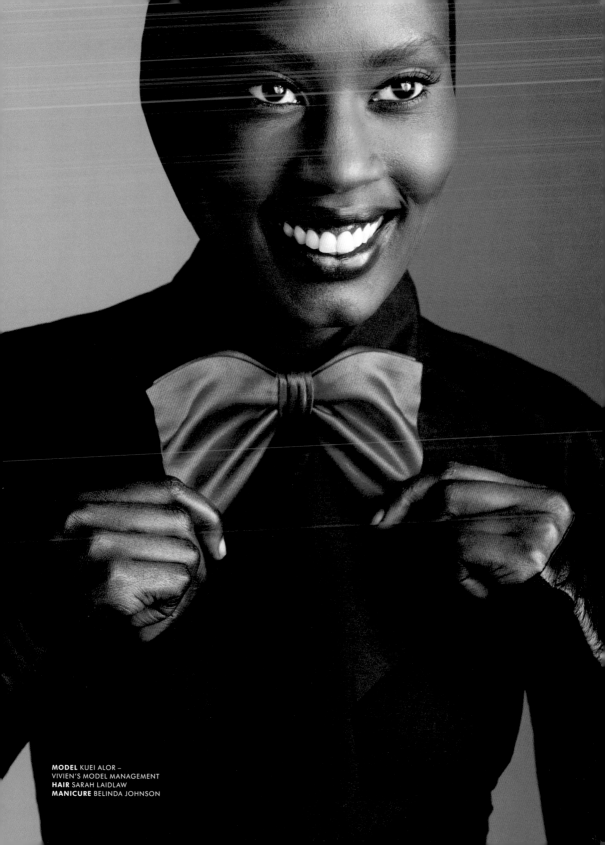

12

NATURALLY SUMPTUOUS

A SOFT BUT GROOMED AND ELEGANT LOOK.

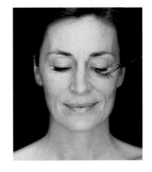

1 LASHES

Curl your lashes, then apply thick mascara to both your top and bottom lashes. Next, add false 3/4 lashes to your top lashes only.

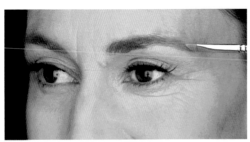

2 SKIN PREP & BROWS

Lightly apply a liquid foundation, and concealer where it's needed, then use a translucent powder all over your face. Define your eyebrows with an angle brush, and you'll see what a difference groomed brows make.

3 CHEEKS & EYELIDS

Use a kabuki brush to apply a soft coral blush high on your cheekbones. Lightly wash this colour over your eyelids, then choose your correct highlighter shade and highlight the inner corners of your eyes and your cupid's bow. Apply a soft berry-pink lipstick.

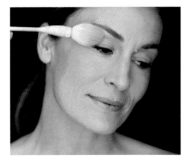

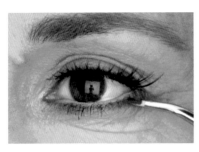

4 EYELINER & PENCIL

Softly apply a brown-black gel eyeliner under your bottom lash line, then a creamy white pencil to the inner rims of each eye before blending it until it looks soft and smudged.

Don't smile when you apply blush, otherwise you'll cause lines.

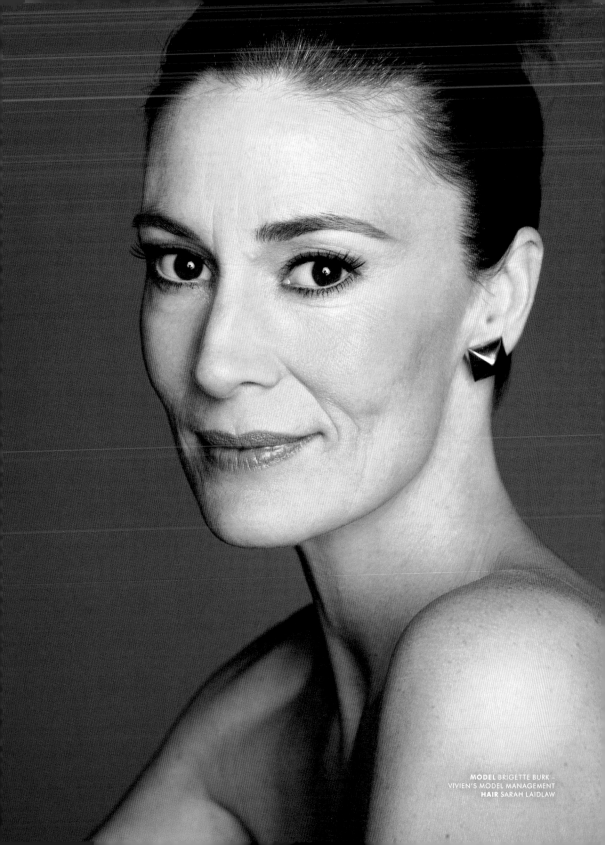

13

KILLER ONYX

AN EASY-TO-APPLY
GRAPHIC EYE THAT
WILL LAST ALL NIGHT.

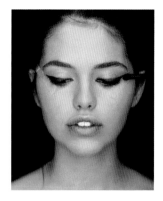

1 EYE SHADOW

Prep your eyes. Following
the natural contour of
your eyes, apply sticky
tape, then lightly brush
matte deep purple eye
shadow along your lash
lines up onto the tape
(for detailed instructions,
see page 67).

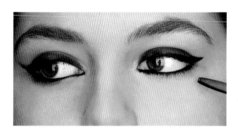

2 EYELINER

Remove the tape, then apply
black kohl pencil to the inner
rim of each eye. Smudge into
the outer corners of each top
lash line.

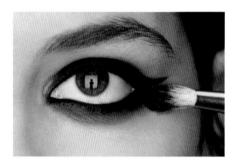

3 EYE SHADOW

Blend a black eye shadow along your
bottom lash lines. If you're having
trouble blending, use some translucent
powder on a clean brush. Clean up any
fallout and apply a cream foundation.

*The inner rim pencil
has a tendency to
fade, so you may
need to reapply this
throughout the day
or night.*

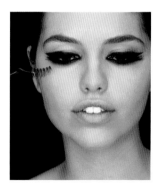

4 LASHES,
CHEEKS & LIPS

Curl your lashes, and
apply lots of black
mascara to your top
and bottom lashes.
Apply false wispy lashes.
Finally, lightly contour
your cheeks, and apply
a clear lip balm.

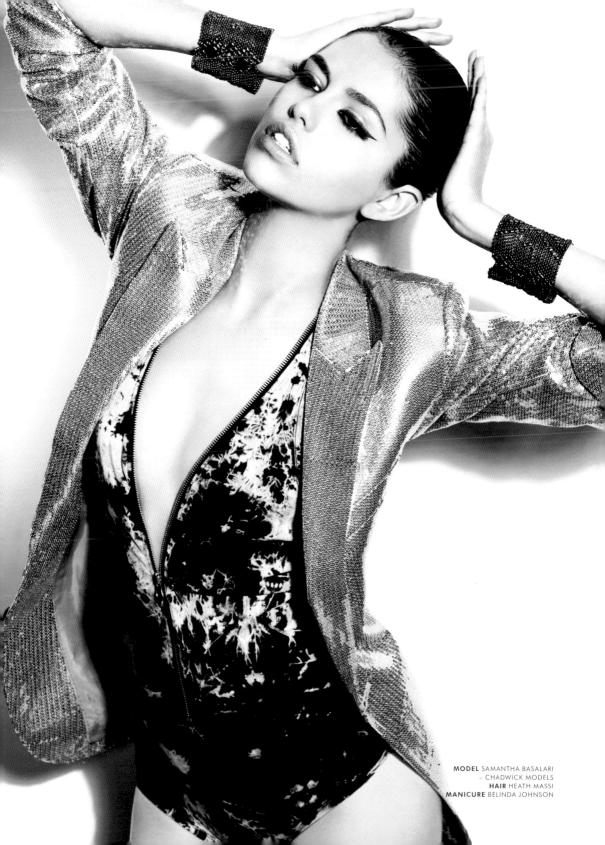

MODEL SAMANTHA BASALARI
– CHADWICK MODELS
HAIR HEATH MASSI
MANICURE BELINDA JOHNSON

14 CRANBERRY KISS

A CLASSIC FEMININE
LOOK THAT WILL
NEVER DATE.

1 EYES, PREP & LIPS

Curl your eyelashes and apply
black mascara. Apply cream
foundation and then bright
red lip pencil all over your lips.

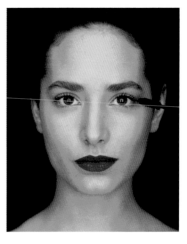

2 EYES, CHEEKS & BROWS

Apply creamy white
pencil to the inner rim
of each eye, and define
your brows. Apply a
soft bronze blush. If
you have time, apply
false 3/4 lashes.

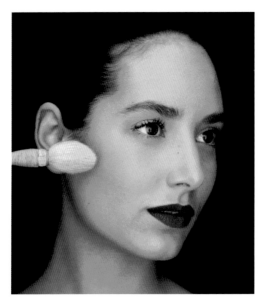

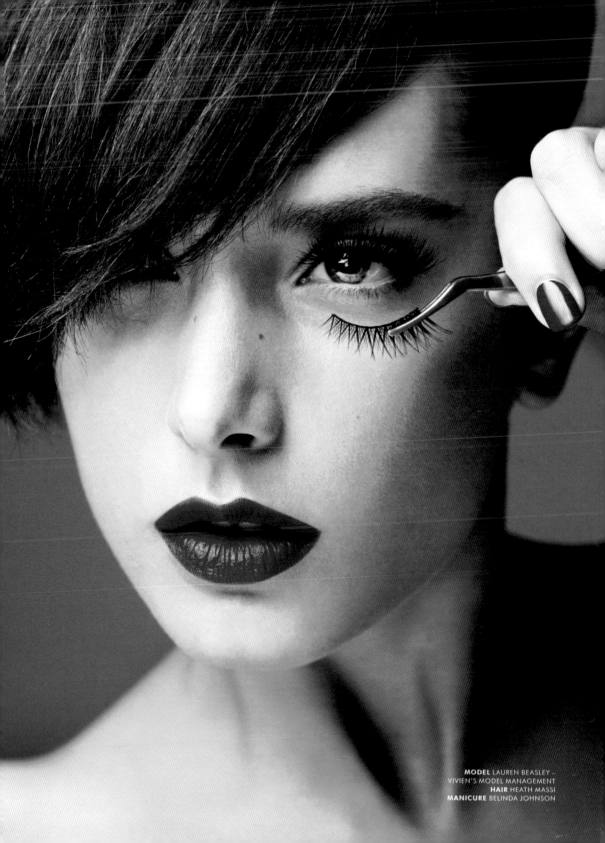

15

GOLDEN MAGNOLIA

REJUVENATE TIRED
SKIN WITH THIS
HOLIDAY GLOW.

1 PREP & EYES

Prep your skin before applying cream
liquid foundation. Then apply a gold
shimmer pigment with a wet brush.
With the same gold colour, highlight
your skin. Take a bronze kohl eye
pencil and smudge along your top
eyelash lines. Use an angled brush
to slightly extend the line outwards.

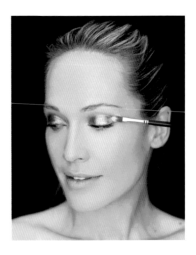

2 LASHES & LIPS

Apply a creamy white pencil to
the inner rims of your eyes. Curl
your lashes, then apply lots of
mascara to your top lashes only.
Finish by applying a rose-tinted
cream blush to your cheeks and
lips. You can add a clear gloss if
you wish.

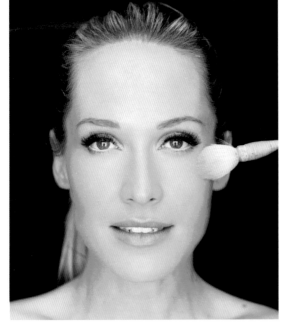

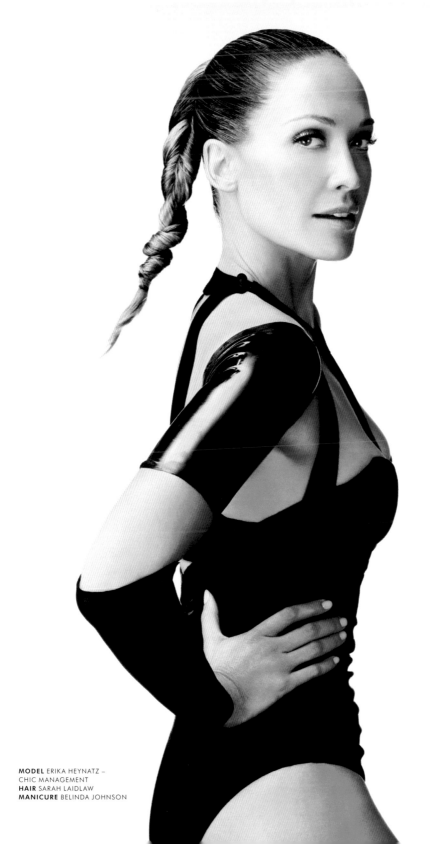

16

VIVA RADIANCE

A QUICK WAY TO LIFT
YOUR EYES AND LOOK
YEARS YOUNGER.

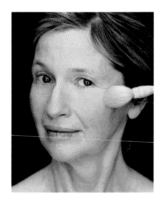

1 FOUNDATION & CHEEKS

Give yourself a healthy
glow by using a rich creamy
foundation before applying
a cream concealer under
your eyes. Then apply
a rose-coloured cream
blush high on your cheeks.
Remember not to smile, or
you'll cause wrinkles.

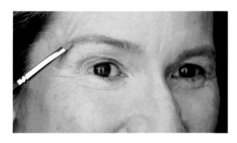

2 BROWS, EYE PREP & LASHES

Define your brows with a brow pencil that matches
your brow hair colour. Powder your lids with
translucent powder. Remember, 99% of your eye
shadow is going to be done looking straight ahead
(see step 3). Curl your lashes.

3 EYE SHADOW

Looking straight into the mirror, colour
in your eyelids with a matte soft grey
eye shadow, as shown, then look down
so you can fill in any gaps you may have
missed. Don't worry about any fallout,
which you can clean up later.

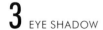

*Never wear a frosty eye
shadow or lipstick, as it
will age you ten years
in an instant.*

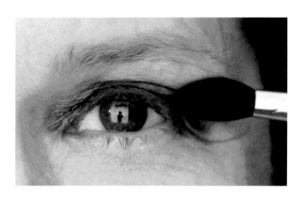

4 LASHES & INNER RIMS

Clean up any fallout with a baby wipe, then use concealer under your eyes. Apply lots of black mascara, adding more to your top lashes. Apply creamy white pencil to the inner rim of each eye.

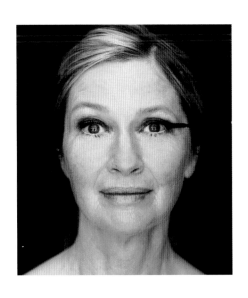

5 CHEEKS & LIPS

If necessary, apply more blush, as it has a tendency to blend into the skin. Use a soft nude lipstick that is closest to your natural lip colour. If your skin is oily or becomes shiny easily, this is a great time to blot it with either a tissue or non-powdered blotting paper before applying light powder. If your skin is dry, however, don't use powder.

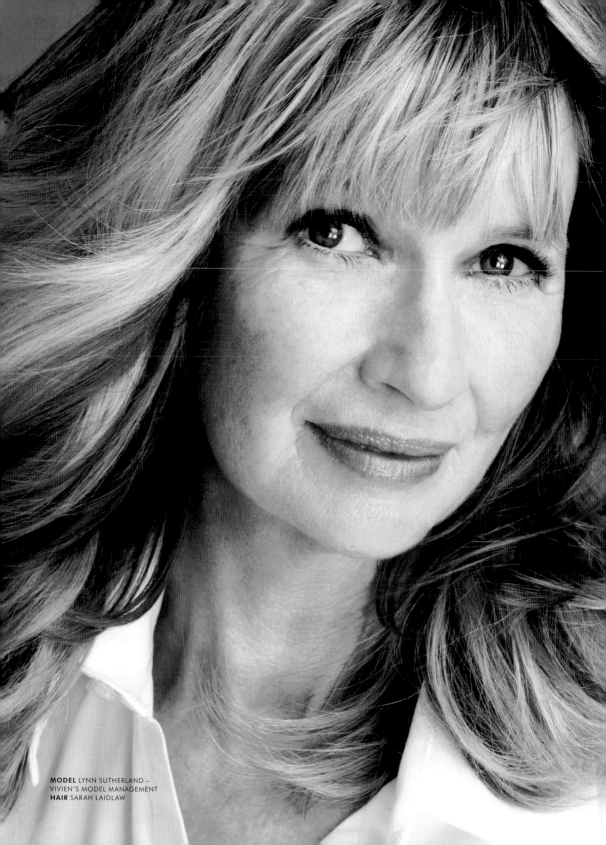

17 | FRESCO CHIC

VOLUPTUOUS
NATURAL LIPS,
THE PERFECT FOIL
FOR A STRONG EYE.

1 PREP & LASHES

Prep your skin, then apply
foundation and concealer.
Apply powder all over,
especially your eyelids.
This gives a velvety finish.
Curl your lashes and apply
mascara, then apply false 3/4
lashes to your top lashes only.

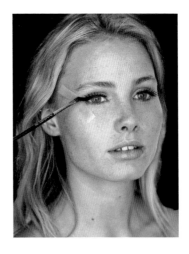

2 EYELINER

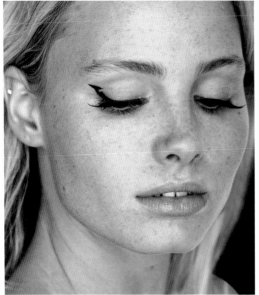

Use sticky tape as a stencil, but stick it to an
item of clothing a few times so it loses some
of its adhesive. Imagine a line running from
the corner of your nose to the outside of
your eye. This is the angle at which to apply
the sticky tape. Trust me, this will lift your
eye. Make sure you apply the eyeliner while
looking straight into the mirror. Use a black
eye shadow, rather than a liquid, because
liquids can crack and look harsh (cream
eyeliners are also a fantastic option).

3 EYELINER

When you look down a little, you'll notice a gap in the eyeliner. That's because you've done the eyeliner looking straight ahead. Fill in the little gap, then continue your liner along your top lash line towards the inner corner of your eye. Repeat for the other eye. Now when you're looking straight ahead, you'll have a perfect eyeliner that lifts your eyes.

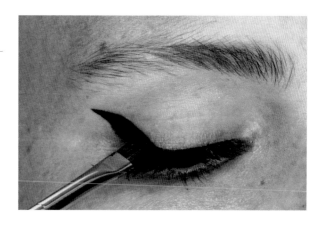

4 CHEEKS, LIPS & LASHES

Contour your cheeks with matte brown eye shadow, but don't apply coloured blush to your cheeks. This darkens under your cheekbones; see the full step-by-step in *Makeup: The Ultimate Guide* (2008), pages 162–7. Matte down your lips with a nude lipstick so they will look fuller and more voluptuous. Lipsticks have more pigment than lip glosses, so they can knock out your natural lip colour, whereas sheer glosses aren't always strong enough. To finish this look, apply lots of mascara to your bottom lashes.

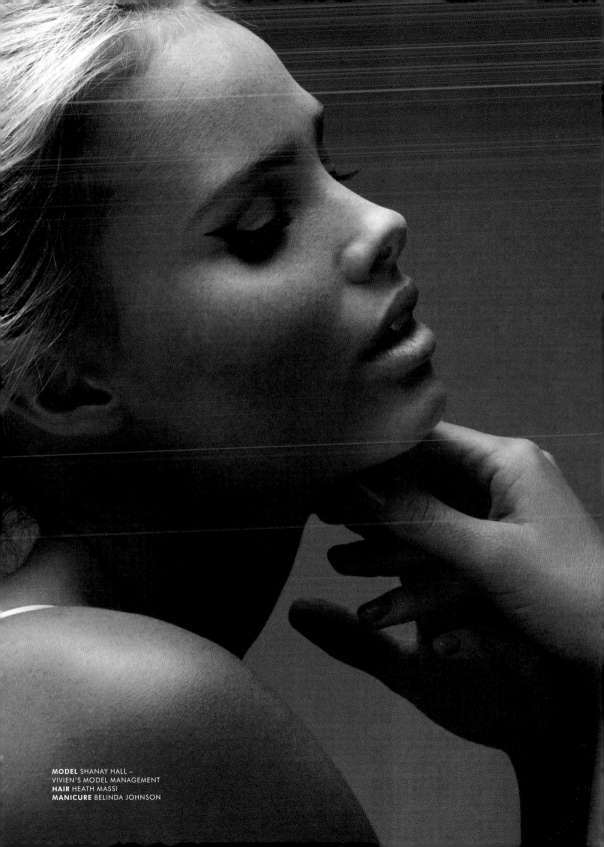

18 TRÈS CHIC

A SOPHISTICATED LOOK FOR STYLISH CITY GIRLS.

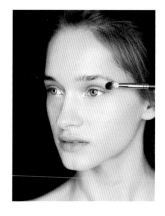

1 SKIN & EYE PREP

Prep your skin, then apply foundation and concealer where required. Powder your eyelids. Do a wash of matte taupe eye shadow across your eyelids.

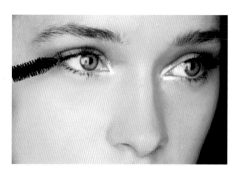

2 INNER RIMS & LASHES

Wet a fine angle brush and apply an intense silver pigment to the inner corners of your eyes. Curl your lashes, then apply lots of mascara to your top and bottom lashes.

3 BROWS, CHEEKS & LIPS

Define your brows. Apply a soft rose-coloured powdered blush. Using your fingertip, and keeping it very soft and sheer, stain your lip with a deep berry- or plum-coloured lipstick.

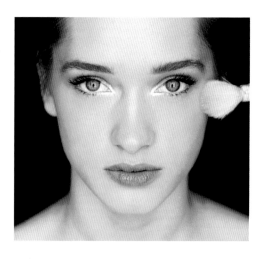

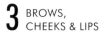

If you never powder your face, make sure you use a cream blush for better blending.

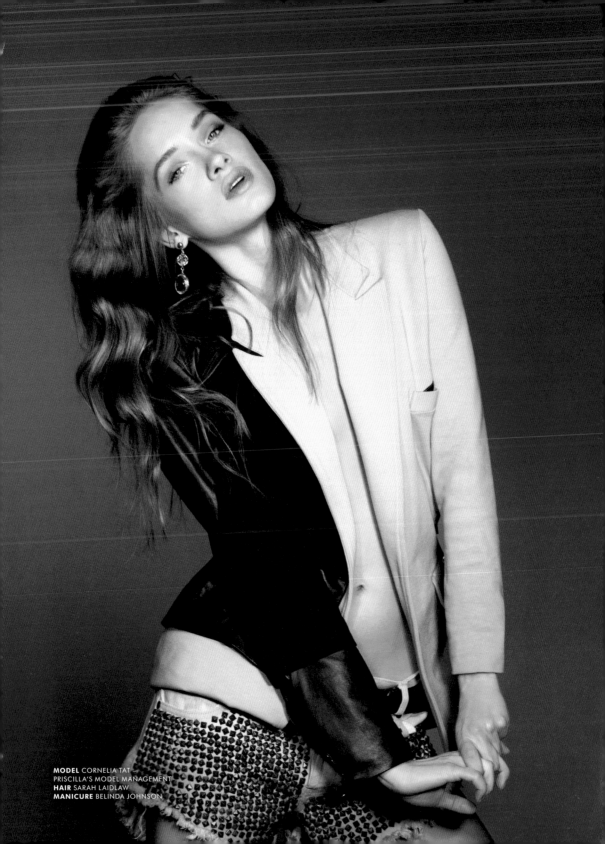

MODEL CORNELIA TAT
PRISCILLA'S MODEL MANAGEMENT
HAIR SARAH LAIDLAW
MANICURE BELINDA JOHNSON

19 | AMETHYST SUPREME

FLATTER BROWN
EYES WITH SOME
AUBERGINE SHADOW.

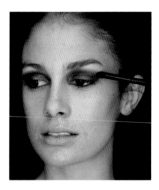

1 DEFINITION & BLENDING

Apply a deep aubergine kohl pencil to your entire eyelid, keeping all the intensity at your lash line. Do the same for the other eye. Apply the same pencil along your inner lower rims. Make sure you blend each eyelid evenly before using a matching eye shadow to blend the edges smoothly.

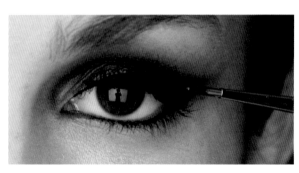

2 LASHES & EYELINER

Curl your lashes, and apply heavy mascara to your top lashes only. Then line your top lash lines with a deep violet liquid eyeliner.

3 BROWS, CHEEKS & LIPS

Clean up any fallout, then apply foundation, or just a bit of concealer if you have great skin. Define your brows, and apply a little deep berry- or plum-coloured lip stain to your cheeks and lips. If your lips are slightly dry, add a hint of clear lip gloss. Highlight your skin if you wish.

If you have a protruding brow bone, then darken that area.

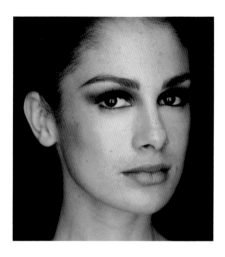

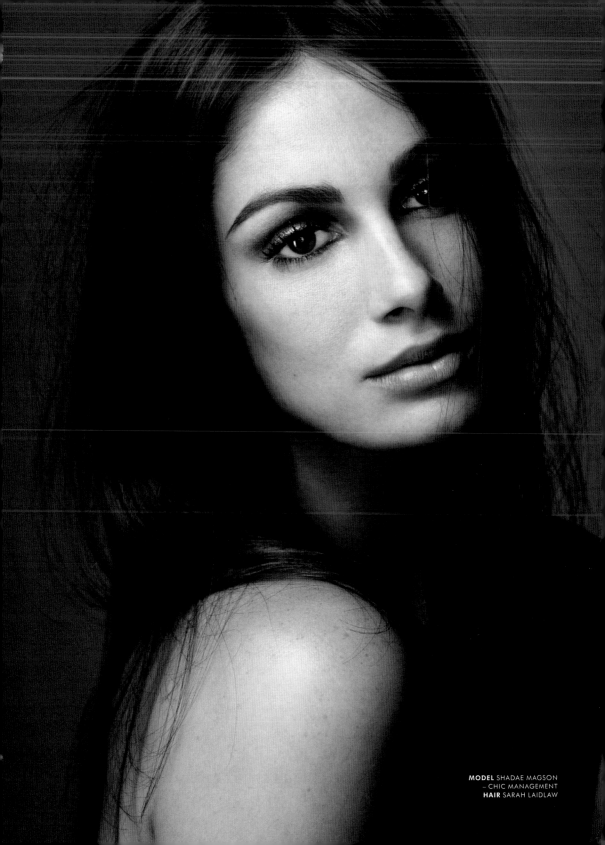

20

ROCK STARLET

A PALE CREAMY LOOK
THAT'S PERFECT FOR
TAWNY BLONDES.

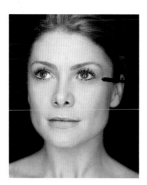

1 PREP, BROWS & LASHES

Prep your skin, then apply liquid foundation and concealer. Powder all over, including your eyelids. I've lightened Natalie's brows with brow mascara, then applied a creamy white pencil to her inner rims. Curl your lashes and apply lots of mascara to your top and bottom lashes.

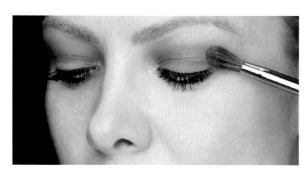

2 EYE SHADOW & BROWS

Apply a soft wash of taupe eye shadow under your eyes and over your entire eyelids, then blend the edges with a light translucent powder. Define your brows.

If you're blonde and want to lighten your eyebrows but don't have a brow mascara, put a little foundation on a clean mascara wand and comb it through.

3 BRONZER & HIGHLIGHTER

Add a soft bronzer, which should be more of a caramel tone than an orange one, to your cheeks. Highlight the inner corners of your eyes and your lips. A soft nude lip works well with this look. If you have an extra five minutes, apply some single lashes.

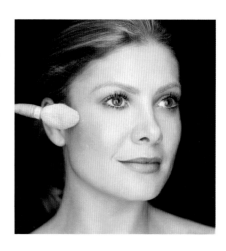

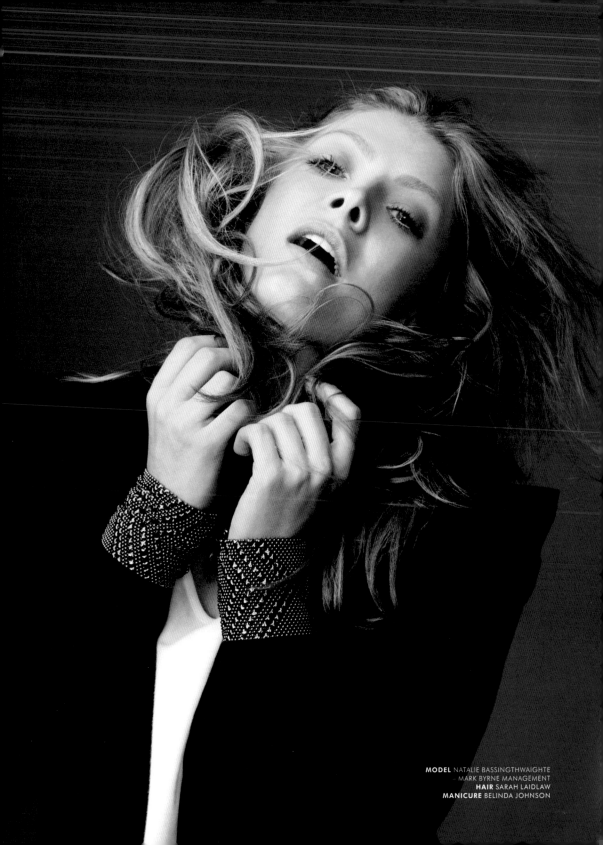

MODEL NATALIE BASSINGTHWAIGHTE
– MARK BYRNE MANAGEMENT
HAIR SARAH LAIDLAW
MANICURE BELINDA JOHNSON

21 | ALLURING PERFECTION

GRACEFUL ELEGANCE
WITH A SOFT
MAHOGANY EYE.

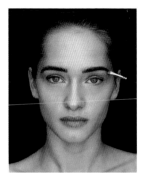

1 EYE PREP & BROWS

Prep your eyelids.
Use concealer where
necessary, and define
your brows with an
angle brush so that you
get full, feathery brows.

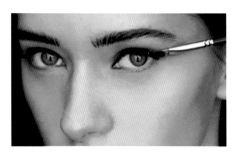

2 LASHES & EYELINER

Curl your lashes, and apply
lots of mascara to your top
lashes only. Using an angle
brush, press a black gel
eyeliner into the lashes
on your top lash lines.

3 UPPER DEFINITION & BLENDING

Looking straight ahead into the mirror,
use a mahogany-brown eye shadow to
follow the natural shape of your brow
bones and extend out. Remember to
blend well.

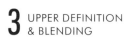

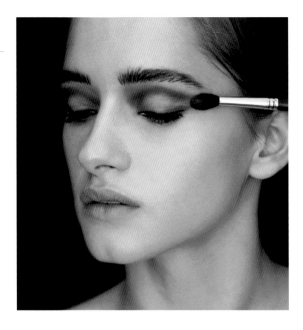

For this look I've applied a few
single eyelashes. You can do
this too, if you have time.
Don't worry if the eyelash
glue is white, as it dries clear.

4 POWDER & KOHL PENCIL

To intensify this look, use liquid black eyeliner and some sticky tape to create a strong black line (see page 67). Peel the tape off. Remove any extra sheen from your face with non-powdered blotting paper, then add a dusting of powder. Generously apply brown kohl pencil to the inner rims of your eyes.

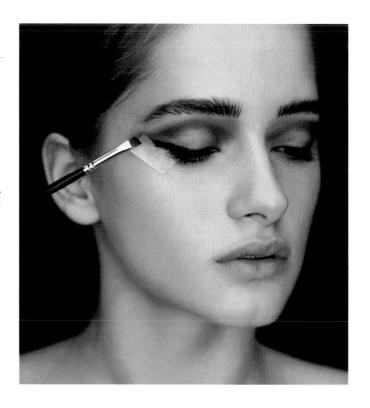

5 LIPS & CHEEKS

Apply just a hint of lip balm. If your lips don't have as much natural colour as the model's, add a little hint of deep berry- or plum-coloured lip stain. Also add a small amount of cream blush.

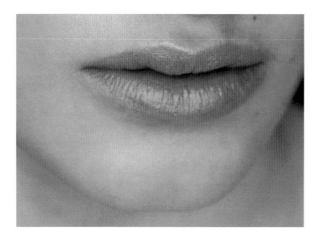

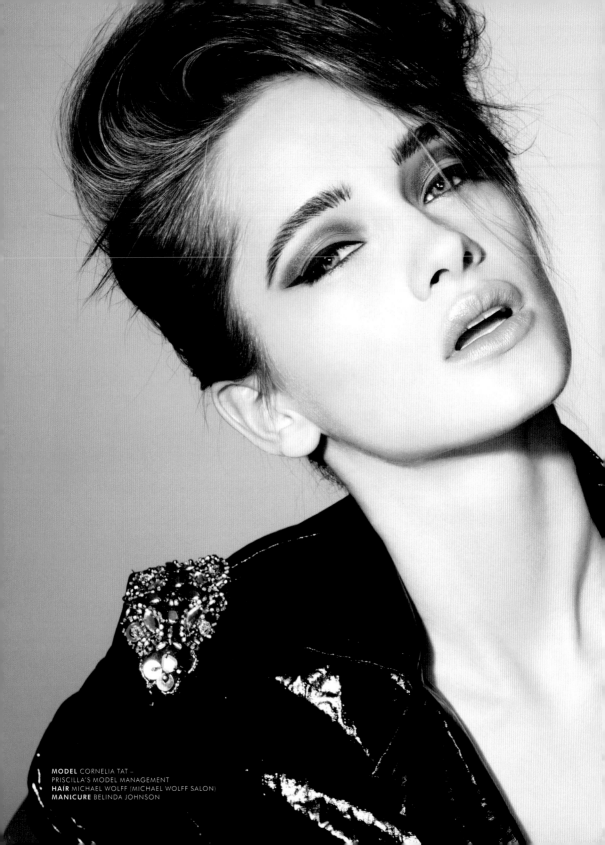

MODEL CORNELIA TAT –
PRISCILLA'S MODEL MANAGEMENT
HAIR MICHAEL WOLFF (MICHAEL WOLFF SALON)
MANICURE BELINDA JOHNSON

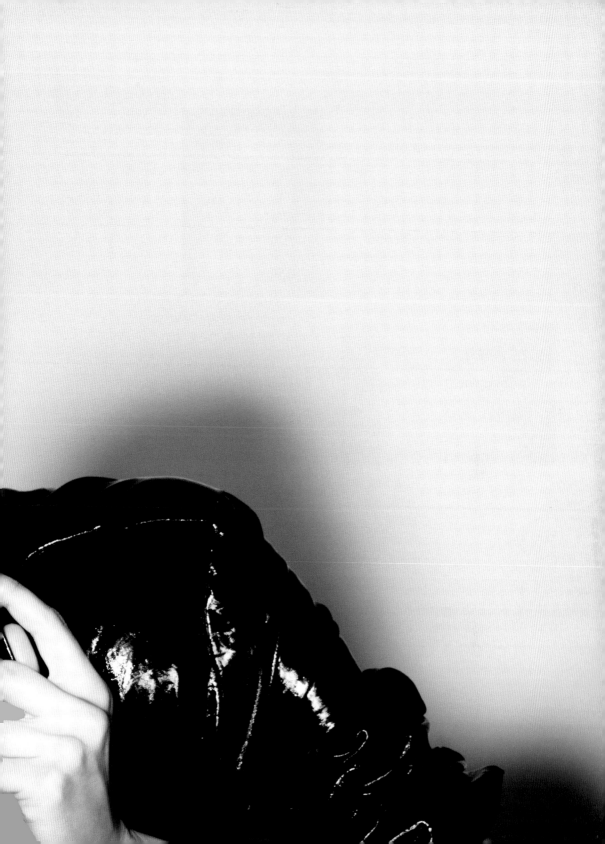

22 | FEMME FATALE

HOLLYWOOD
GLAMOUR FOR
DRAMA QUEENS.

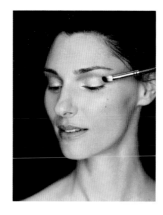

1 PREP, PIGMENT & EYE SHADOW

Prep your skin
and apply cream
foundation. Add a soft
wash of gold pigment
to your eyelids, then
a matte taupe eye
shadow just under your
brow bones. Highlight
the inner corners with
a silver pigment.

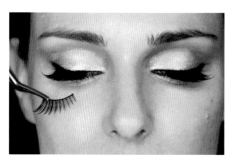

2 EYELINER & LASHES

Use an angle brush to lightly smudge black
gel eyeliner along your top lash lines.
Curl your lashes, and apply lots of black
mascara to your top lashes only. Apply
false 3/4 lashes. In this shot I've already
applied the lashes and I'm holding up
another one so you can see the lash type.

3 POWDER, CHEEKS & LIPS

Apply translucent powder over your
whole face, then apply a creamy white
pencil to the lower inner rim of each
eye. Apply a dark burgundy lipstick,
then a very soft rose-coloured blush to
your cheeks. With a dark nail polish, this
is a strong look that makes a statement.

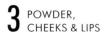

*Only use the silver pigment
if it suits your eye colour;
if not, stick to the gold.*

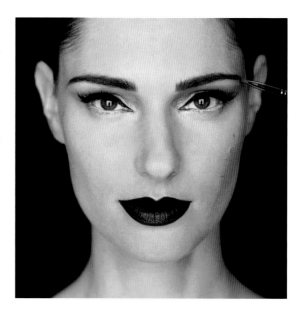

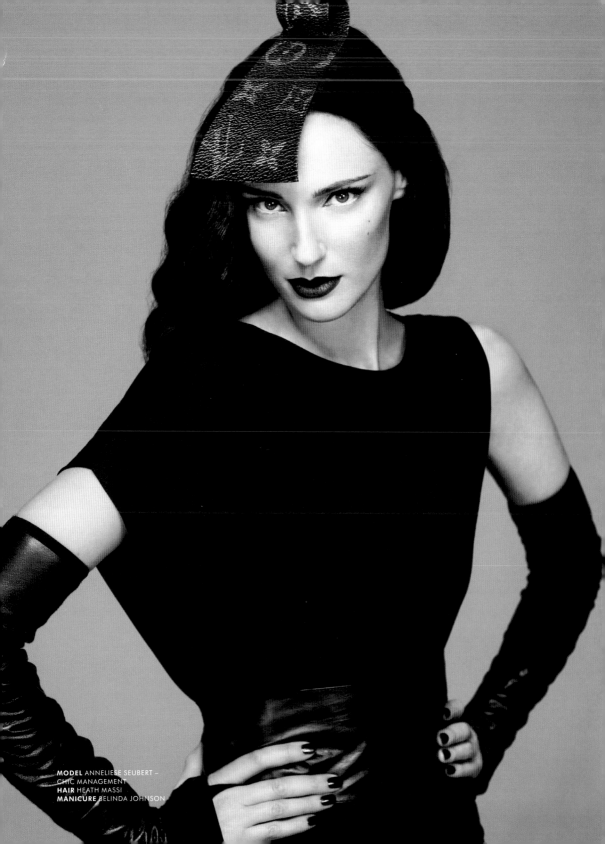

MODEL ANNELIESE SEUBERT –
CHIC MANAGEMENT
HAIR HEATH MASSI
MANICURE BELINDA JOHNSON

23 | MOD GLOSS

A STRONGLY DEFINED EYE WITH A FLASH OF SILVER.

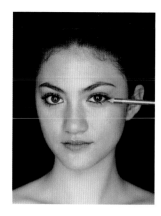

1 EYE PREP, KOHL & LASHES

If your skin is clear, prep your eyes only. Line the inner rim of your eye and the end of the bottom lash line with a metallic silver kohl pencil. Repeat for the other eye. Curl your lashes and apply lots of mascara to your top and bottom lashes.

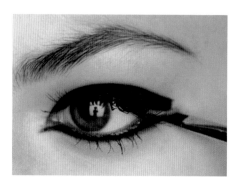

2 EYELINER & BLENDING

Keeping the shape quite square, apply black liquid eyeliner straight across your top lids. Wait for it to dry, then take the same eyeliner along the bottom eyelash line, flicking it out along the edge. Use a sharp angle brush for precision.

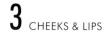

3 CHEEKS & LIPS

Apply a rosy pink cream blush and a nude matte lipstick. You can use a lip pencil as lipstick here, but make sure you colour in your whole lip.

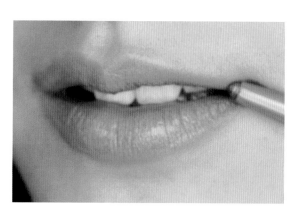

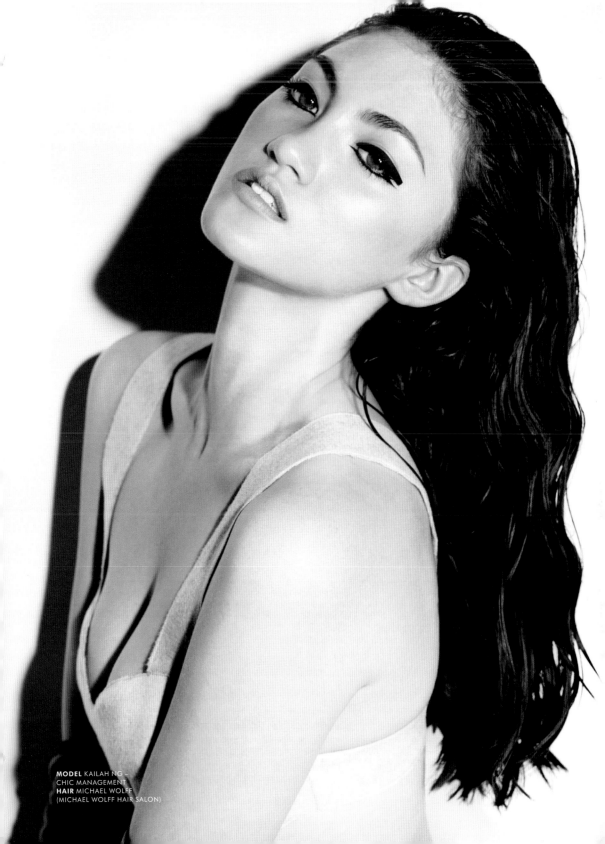

24 | ORCHID SMILE

A FRESH GLAMOROUS LOOK WITH SWISH SHIMMERY HIGHLIGHTS.

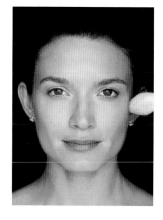

1 PREP, POWDER & CHEEKS

Apply foundation, and concealer where required. Powder all over, then apply a bright tangerine orange blush to your cheeks. The model has fabulous skin, so I've used a shimmery blush, but if you're conscious of fine lines around your eyes, keep the blush matte.

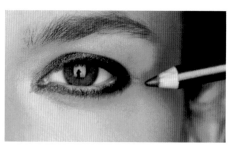

2 DEFINITION

Take a chocolate-brown eye pencil and smudge it around your whole eye. Don't worry if it looks a little rough—it just needs to heat up on your skin for a minute so it becomes easier to smudge. Repeat for the other eye.

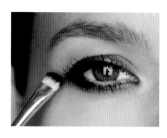

3 LASHES

Use a mini square blending brush to smudge that pencil and extend the edges. Curl your lashes and apply lots of mascara to your top and bottom lashes.

4 LIPS & BROWS

Finish off with a bright orange matte lipstick. Wet your brush, then add shimmery gold pigment to the inner corners of your eyes. Finally, lightly define your brows.

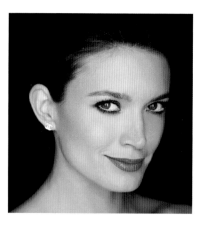

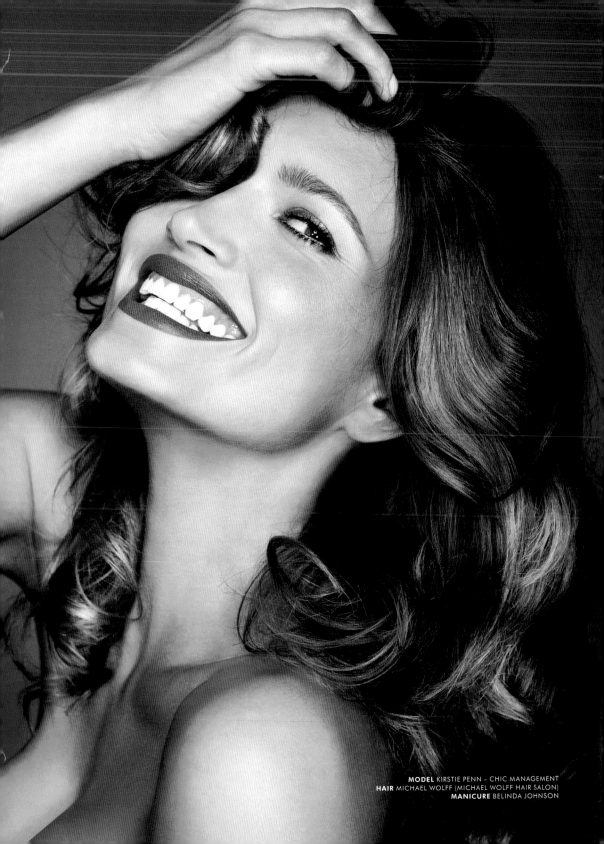

25 EXQUISITE DEFINITION

SUMMON YOUR INNER
ROCK CHICK WITH SMOKY
EYES AND NUDE LIPS.

1 EYE PREP

Because this look requires
soft, smoky eyes, just apply
sheer liquid foundation, then
lightly powder your eyelids
so you can blend perfectly.

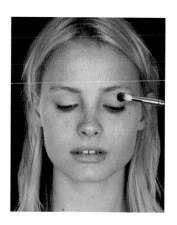

2 EYE SHADOW

With a medium eye shadow brush, apply
a soft, matte grey eye shadow along your
entire eyelids, stopping under your brow
bones. If you have trouble blending your
eye shadow, pick up translucent powder
with a clean brush and use it to blend.

3 LOWER DEFINITION

Use a medium-sized brush to
apply the same colour under
your eyes, then use an angle
brush to apply a darker shade
of grey along the lash line.

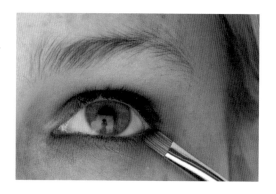

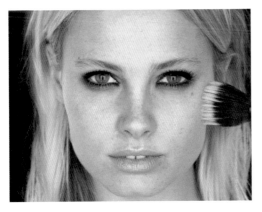

4 EYES, LASHES & HIGHLIGHTER

Apply a black kohl pencil along your top and bottom lash lines, then softly smudge with a small eye shadow brush. Curl your lashes, apply lots of black mascara to your top and bottom lashes and clean up any fallout. Use sheer liquid foundation mixed with luminiser to highlight your skin all over.

5 CHEEKS

Conceal any blemishes. Using a kabuki brush, apply cream blush high on your cheeks. Don't smile as you apply blush, or you'll create lines.

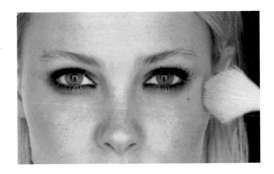

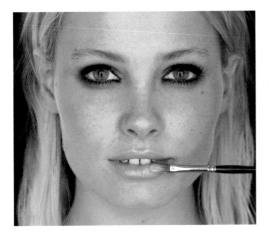

6 LIPS

This look is great with just a little bit of lip balm, but you can even out your lips with a nude lipstick.

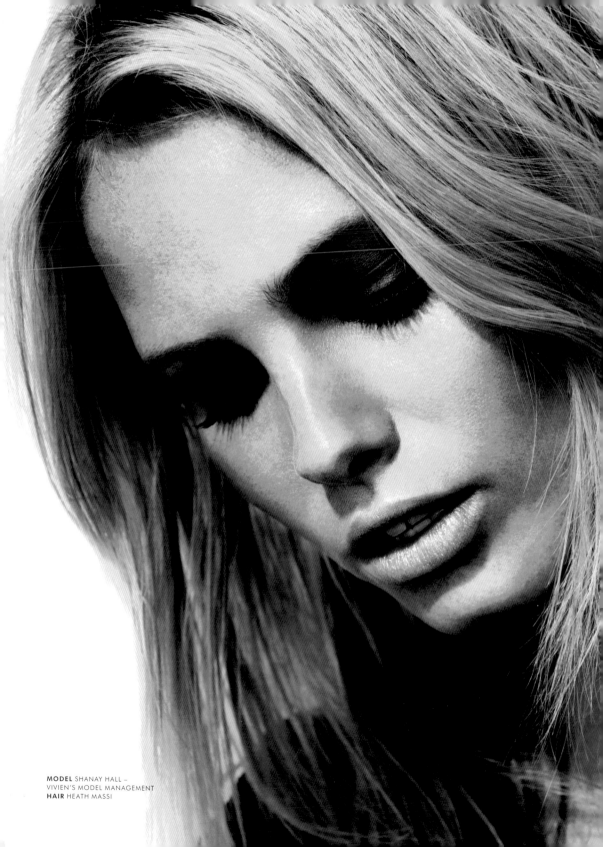

INDEX

Acknowledgments

A huge thank you to all the people who've made this book possible.

Steven Chee, photographer; Geoffrey Burger Nolan, stylist; Stephen Smedley, designer; Grace Testa, retoucher; and Bronwyn Fraser, colour expert. My literary agents Mark Byrne and Lisa Hanrahan; my publisher Louise Thurtell and editor Sarah Baker; and the incredible Kate Hyde.

Tobias Rowles, digital operator; Duncan Pickett, photographic assistant; makeup assistants Lei Tai, Kathy Criniti, Casey Gore, Gina Guirguis and Michael Shiailis; Elena Gomez, typist; Phaedra Giblin, typist/makeup assistant; and Katherine Teroxy, Geoffrey Burger Nolan's assistant. Hair stylists Heath Massi, Sarah Laidlaw, Michael Wolff (Michael Wolff Hair Salon), Joel Phillips; manicurist Belinda Johnson; and Cameron Jane, Samantha Robinson and Flor Sepulveda, Cameron Jane Makeup School.

At Chic Management – Ursula Hufnagl and Yonta Taiwo, and models Lizzy B, Cassi Colvin, Erika Heynatz, Catherine McNeil, Shadae Magson, Kailah Ng, Kirstie Penn, Anneliese Seubert, Sarah Stephens and Kieta Van Ewyk. At Priscilla's Model Management – Jaz Daly, and models Chrystal Copland, Kerry Doyle, Georgia Fowler, Caitlin Lomax, Eve Lui, Tina Malou and Cornelia Tat. At Vivien's Model Management – Susie Deveridge and Tineke Dickson, and models Kuei Alor, Lauren Beasley, Brigette Burk, Rachael Grasso, Shanay Hall and Lynn Sutherland. At Chadwick Models – Sarah Grant, and model Samantha Basalari.

Natalie Bassingthwaighte – Mark Byrne Management.

Wendy Tomaino – Smiink Eyelashes and Ultimate Brush Roll. DLM; Luxe Studios; The Front for supplying extra lights and equipment; Juliet Fallowfield and Amelia – Chanel; Kenneth Beck – www.carbon8.com.au.

Fashion credits

Items not listed are stylist's own. **ii, 3** and **69** Clothes: Christopher Esber. **vi and 63** Bodysuit: This is Genevieve; Arm bands: Suzy O'Rourke. **6 top** Ring: Vintage. **6 bottom** Headpiece: Suzy O'Rourke; Flowered jumpsuit: Billion Dollar Babes. **7** Jewellery: Kerry Rocks. **34** Tank top: Nathan Smith; White boy pants: Holeproof; Necklace: Christian Dior. **37** Necklace, black bracelet and round ring: Chanel; Small ring, round bracelets and earrings: Peep Toe. **39** Tank top: Nathan Smith. **41** Tank top: Nathan Smith. **45** All-in-one: Billion Dollar Babes; Hat: Suzy O'Rourke; Rubber gloves: Reactor. **51** All clothing: Chanel. **53** Dress and top: Alistair Trung. **55** Black button shirt: Christopher Esber; Black skull cap: Suzy O'Rourke; Gloves: Alistair Trung; Bowtie: World. **59** Bodysuit: Evil Twin; Jacket: Jack London; Bracelets: Diva. **66** White shirt: Alistair Trung. **71** Jacket (beige): Sara Phillips; Jacket (black): Christopher Esber; Studded denim shorts: One Teaspoon. **75** White top: Mink Pink; Necklaces: Christian Dior; Cuffs: Diva; Jacket: Manning Cartell. **78–9** Jacket: Tim O'Connor; Shoulder adornment: Headband by Diva. **81** Dress: Christopher Esber; Belt and gauntlets: Alistair Trung; Paper accessory concept: Geoffrey Burger Nolan. **83** Gloves: Alistair Trung. **88** Clothes: Christopher Esber.